# A Casebook of Electrocardiographic Tracings

Jorge I. Martinez-Lopez
Stephen P. Glasser
Pamela I. Clark

**John Wright • PSG Inc**
*Boston Bristol London*
1982

Library of Congress Cataloging in Publication Data
Main entry under title:

A casebook of electrocardiographic tracings.

Bibliography: p.
Includes index.
1. Electrocardiography--Case studies.
I. Martinez-Lopez, Jorge I., 1926-
II. Glasser, Stephen P. III. Clark, Pamela I.
[DNLM: 1. Electrocardiography--Case studies.
2. Heart diseases--Diagnosis--Case studies. WG 140
N3855c]
RC683.5.E5C26 616.1'207547 81-16115
ISBN 0-88416-307-5 AACR2

Published by:
John Wright • PSG Inc, 545 Great Road, Littleton,
Massachusetts 01460, U.S.A.
John Wright & Sons Ltd, 42–44 Triangle West,
Bristol BS8 1EX, England

Medicine is an ever-changing science. As new research and clinical experience broaden our knowledge, changes in treatment and drug therapy are required. The editor and the publisher of this work have made every effort to ensure that the treatment and drug dosage schedules herein are accurate and in accord with the standards accepted at the time of publication. Readers are advised, however, to check the product information sheet included in the package of each drug they plan to administer to be certain that changes have not been made in the recommended dose or in the indications and contraindications for administration. This recommendation is of particular importance in regard to new or infrequently used drugs.



Printed in the United States of America.

International Standard Book Number: 0-88416-307-5

Library of Congress Catalog Card Number: 81-16115

Dedicated to Richard Ashman, PhD and
Louis Levy, II, MD

# Contributors

Karen Bowyer, MD
Former Resident
Department of Internal Medicine
University of South Florida College of Medicine
Tampa, Florida

Pamela I. Clark, RN
Assistant Professor of Medicine
Supervisor, Cardiac Non Invasive Laboratories
University of South Florida College of Medicine
The James A. Haley Veterans Administration Hospital
Tampa, Florida

Stephen P. Glasser, MD, FACC, FACP
Professor of Medicine
Director, Division of Cardiovascular Medicine
Director, Cardiac Non Invasive Laboratories
The James A. Haley Veterans Administration Hospital
Medical Director, Tampa Bay Cardiac Prevention and Rehabilitation Program
Tampa, Florida

Jorge I. Martinez-Lopez, MD, FACC, FACP, FCCP
Professor of Medicine (Cardiology)
Department of Medicine
LSU Medical Center
Director, Cardiology Department
Charity Hospital of Louisiana
New Orleans, Louisiana

Mallan G. Morgan, MD
Former Cardiology Fellow and Clinical Associate in Medicine
LSU School of Medicine in Shreveport
Shreveport, Louisiana

# Contents

# Preface

This book is an outgrowth of efforts initiated by the American Heart Association-Louisiana in 1975. Prior to that date, the Journal of the Louisiana State Medical Society published an ECG monthly and a very brief interpretation. One of us (JML) approached Dr. Norton W. Voorhies, editor of the section, and suggested expanding the objective of the section, under the aegis of the AHA-LA, to provide more of an educational experience for the readers. Dr. Voorhies won the approval of the Editorial Board to do this, and it fell on our shoulders to provide the scientific essays.

To entice the subscribers of the Journal to read the material in the section, we decided to utilize titles that would pique their curiosity, rather than to use the traditional titles which give away the contents of the essays. The format was simple. Titles were to provide a subtle clue that could be used in approaching the interpretation of the tracings. In the pages which followed the tracing, the electrocardiographic diagnosis and the elucidation of the interpretation were given. That concluded, a brief discussion followed, and selected bibliographic references were given.

Judging by the comments reaching us, we believe our goal of making the section infomative and educational was reached. Later, it was suggested that we compile our presentations into the volume you now have.

The publishers, John Wright • PSG, reviewed some of the manuscripts and concurred with the idea. The Editorial Board of the Journal of the Louisiana State Medical Society gave us permission to pursue this endeavor.

This volume is by no means encyclopedic, nor are the bibliographic references extensive, but those listed are key references. The book does not cover basics of ECG interpretation for it is not intended for the neophyte, but rather it is directed at individuals who already have a basic knowledge of electrocardiography and who wish to expand their horizons further.

The reader is therefore encouraged to read titles carefully, to examine each tracing carefully, and, once he has decided on the electrocardiographic diagnosis, to turn the page and digest the information which follows. If we can evoke your curiosity and your interest in each article, the material provided in the discussion should stimulate you to read more and in detail.

At the conclusion of the book a total of 50 questions is provided. The publishers, ever cognizant of the current trends in Continuing Medical Education, suggested that these be appended for those interested in obtaining CME credits. Instructions are included with the questions.

We are grateful to those who encouraged us in this endeavor. Generating these monthly articles for the Journal was a challenge, as well as a refreshing experience. Our thanks go to the American Heart Association-Louisiana, to the Editorial Board of the Journal of the Louisiana State Medical Society, and in particular to Dr. Norton W. Voorhies, who has been our most avid supporter. And we are especially indebted to Ms. Jane Baudoin and Ms. Carol Bazer for secretarial assistance, and to Ms. Lisa Candelaria for the clarity of the reproductions.

Jorge I. Martinez-Lopez
Stephen P. Glasser
Pamela I. Clark

## NUMBER 1 *"Q" Me In* Jorge I. Martinez-Lopez

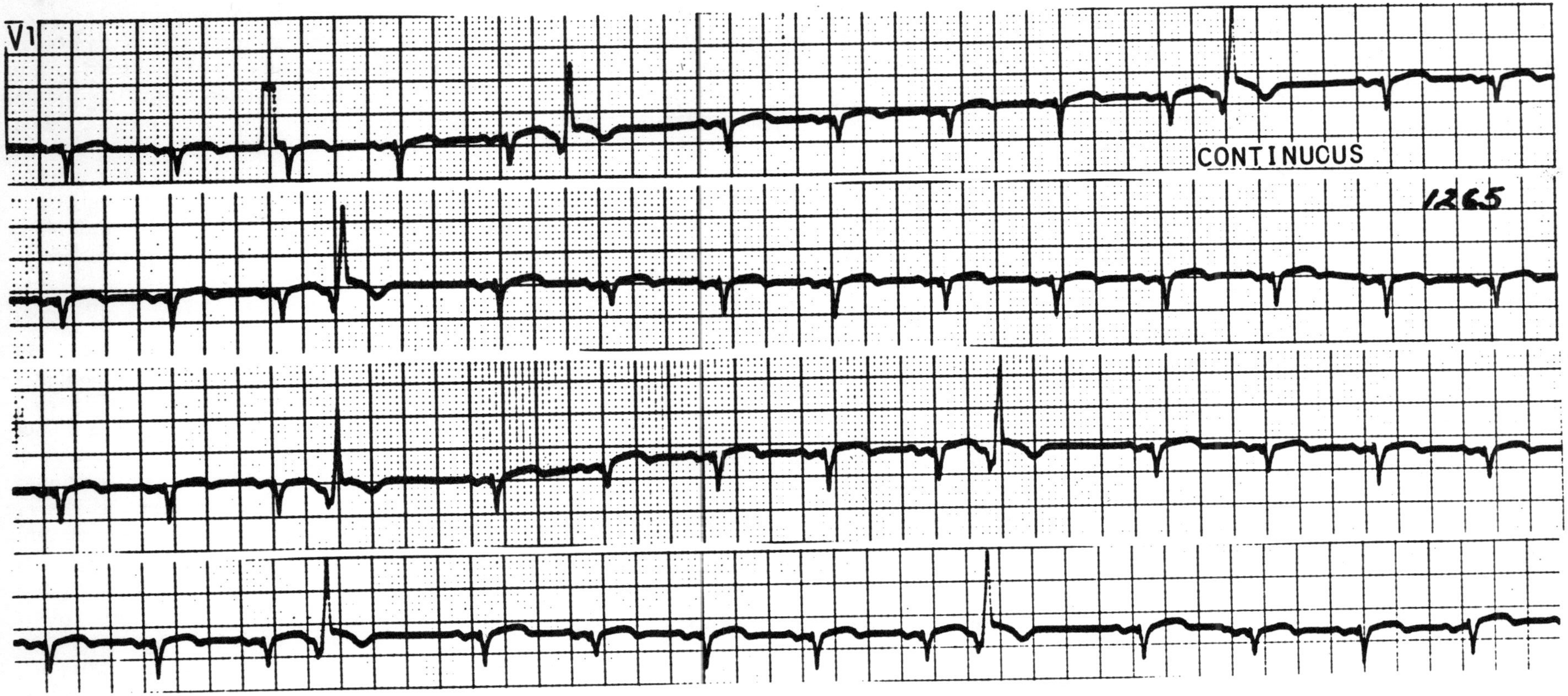


**Figure 1** No clinical data are available on the tracing shown, taken in a 56-year-old man.

# NUMBER 1 *"Q" Me In* Jorge I. Martinez-Lopez

## ELUCIDATION

**Diagnosis—***"Infarct-pattern" ventricular premature impulses*

Normal sinus rhythm is present. All intervals in the dominant rhythm (PR, QRS and QT) are normal in duration. The terminal negativity in the P waves suggests atrial pathology.

Trigeminy is noted, consisting of two normally conducted sinus impulses and a ventricular premature impulse. This trio would not be so interesting if it were not for the following facts. First, ventricular premature impulses (VPI) have *long* fixed coupling intervals (post-mature). Because there is concomitant sinus arrhythmia, portions of the P wave deform the initial part of the last two VPI in the lower strip. Second, the VPI show deep Q waves (QR), slight elevation of the ST segment, and inverted T waves. Such VPI are designated as *"infarct-pattern"* VPI.

## DISCUSSION

*Normal* Q waves occur in most electrocardiographic tracings, especially in the lateral precordial leads, and represent the initial left-to-right depolarization of the interventricular septum. *Abnormal* Q waves are defined as being deep in proportion to the R wave (Q/R amplitude ratio greater than 25%), or lasting longer than 0.03 or 0.04 second, or a combination of both, depending on the lead.

Abnormal Q waves are considered essential for the electrocardiographic diagnosis of recent or remote myocardial infarction. Similar changes, however, can develop transiently during episodes of angina pectoris or coronary insufficiency, and disappear after cessation of the attack. On occasion, abnormal Q waves can be seen in tracings from patients *without* coronary artery disease. A few examples include IHSS, WPW syndrome, pulmonary embolism, infiltrative disorders of the myocardium, and primary myocardial disease.

Electrocardiographic evidence of myocardial infarction is persistent in the majority of cases but it can become masked sometimes. This can occur through spontaneous "normalization" of the abnormal Q waves over a period of time, by the subsequent development of hemiblocks or bundle branch block, or by permanent ventricular pacing. Unless previous tracings show the abnormal Q waves, the diagnosis of myocardial infarction may go unrecognized.

In 1943, Dressler reported the "unmasking" of an acute inferior wall infarction by uniform ventricular premature impulses (VPI) in a patient with left bundle branch block. This interesting phenomenon, briefly discussed below, may be more frequently encountered if physicians are made aware of it.

VPI are of common occurrence in the adult population; their significance is determined by a variety of coexisting factors. They may represent an electrophysiologic event of no pathological significance or may be a manifestation of a serious underlying disorder, drug toxicity, or both. Ominous implications have been attributed to their prematurity, to their quantitative frequency, and to whether they are uniform or multiform, right or left ventricular in origin, etc.

Little attention has consistently been given to the presence or absence of abnormal Q waves in VPI. Bisteni and co-workers stressed the importance of analyzing isolated VPI in confirming the diagnosis of myocardial infarction. Experimentally, right and left VPI were produced mechanically in dogs before and after ligation of the left anterior descending coronary artery. Only after the infarction was produced did the VPI demonstrate a QR pattern (QR, QRs, Qrs complexes) in leads reflecting potential variations of the ventricles; aVr and aVl were of no value. Their clinical observations, and those reported by others, were in agreement with the experimental findings.

"Infarct-pattern" VPI can occur in three different settings. *First,* the abnormal Q wave is displayed in both the dominant rhythm and in the VPI in the same lead. Since both QRS complexes show the infarct pattern, there is nothing to unmask. *Second,* the abnormal Q wave is seen only in the VPI but not in the QRS complexes of the dominant rhythm in the same lead; this represents "unmasking." This pattern can also occur in 8% to 9% of tracings from apparently normal subjects (false positives). *Third,* abnormal Q waves are present in the ventricular complexes of the dominant rhythm and absent in the VPI in the same lead, but present in other leads, ie, VPI fail to show features of infarction. The incidence of these so-called "false negatives" is approximately 30%.

In conclusion, the diagnosis and localization of *concealed* myocardial infarction can be made with significant degree of accuracy by careful analysis of uniform VPI; specifically, when the ventricular complexes of the dominant rhythm do not show abnormal Q waves but the VPI do. If, in addition, the ST segment is elevated and the T wave inverted, the diagnosis of *concealed acute* myocardial infarction can be made with confidence. Correlation of the "infarct-pattern" VPI with the history and the clinical findings is essential if this method is to remain useful, since both false positives and false negatives do occur.

## SELECTED READINGS


Benchimol A, Lasry JE, Carvalho FR: The ventricular premature contraction. Its place in the diagnosis of ischemic heart disease. *Am Heart J* 65:334, 1963.

Bisteni A, Medrano GA, Sodi-Pallares D: Ventricular premature beats in the diagnosis of myocardial infarction. *Br Heart J* 23:521, 1961.

Dressler W: A case of myocardial infarction masked by bundle branch block but revealed by occasional premature ventricular beats. *Am J Med Sci* 206:36, 1943.

Silverman JJ, Salomon S: Myocardial infarction pattern disclosed by ventricular extrasystoles. *Am J Cardiol* 4:695, 1959.

Szilagyi N, Ginsburg M: Acute myocardial infarction revealed in the presence of right bundle branch block and ventricular extrasystoles. *Am J Cardiol* 9:632, 1962.

## NUMBER 2 *VVO, VVT, or VAT?* Jorge I. Martinez-Lopez

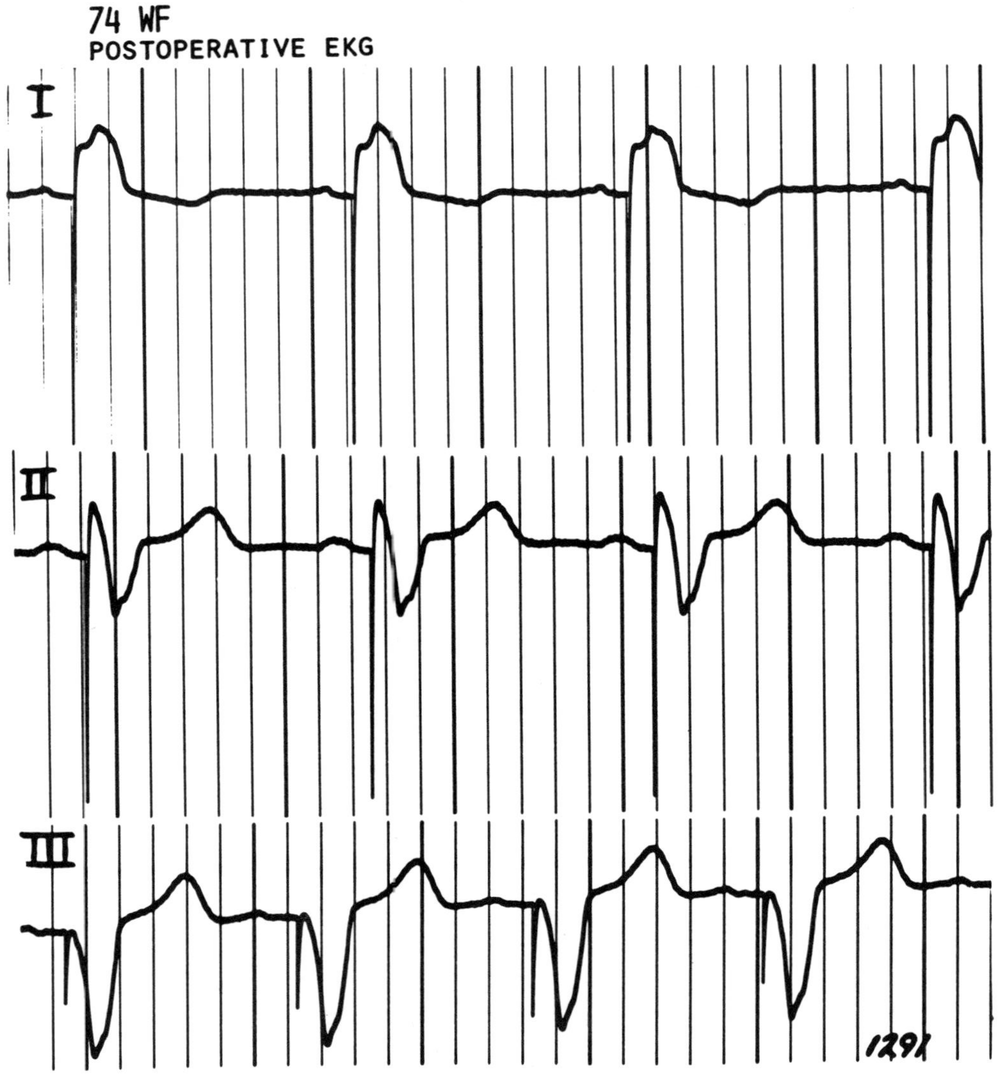


**Figure 2** This three-bipolar limb-lead tracing was recorded postoperatively in a 74-year-old woman. She had been admitted because of dizziness and near-syncopal episodes.

# NUMBER 2 *VVO, VVT, or VAT?* Jorge I. Martinez-Lopez

## ELUCIDATION

**Diagnosis**—*P-wave synchronized pacemaker*

Sinus P waves are present in the three leads recorded simultaneously; they have a constant temporal relationship.

The QRS complexes are broad and abnormal in duration, and are associated with secondary ST-T wave changes. The mean QRS vector is deviated abnormally to the left.

Prominently displayed in all leads are pacemaker spikes, following every P wave and preceding every QRS; they are negatively oriented.

## DISCUSSION

The patient was found to have bilateral bundle branch block with variable degree of AV block and long pauses. Electrophysiologic studies showed the block to occur below the bundle of His. Sinoatrial function was found to be intact. Accordingly, it was decided to implant a P-wave synchronized pacemaker.*

Early artificial cardiac pacemakers were *asynchronous* or *competitive*. Because they discharged at a fixed rate, pacing impulses fell at random in the cardiac cycle. Though popular at first, they gained notoriety for their ability to induce ventricular fibrillation and sudden death when the pacemaker stimulus fell during the vulnerable period of the ventricles. As a consequence, *synchronous* or *noncompetitive* modes were then developed to circumvent this possibility and to prevent other arrhythmias induced by competitive pacemakers; they are now favored. *Noncompetitive* or synchronous pacemakers currently in use are: ventricular inhibited, ventricular triggered, AV sequential, and the P-wave (atrial) synchronous.

The *P-wave synchronous pacemaker* consists of a power generator and two electrode leads. One electrode lead is placed in the right atrium by the pervenous route, and the other in the right ventricle. The atrial lead is designed to sense the P wave of the ECG, when present. Sensing is then relayed to the timing mechanism within the generator so that, after a delay corresponding to the natural AV delay, the pacing impulse is delivered to the ventricle via the second lead. In this manner, the atrioventricular activation sequence and atrial contribution to ventricular filling are maintained. The output rate of the pacemaker can be programmed externally, ie, skin penetration is not required.

Equally important is the fact that the ventricular rate will vary in response to changes in SA node firing at rest and with exertional activities. However, to prevent exceedingly fast or slow ventricular rates in response to fast or slow supraventricular rhythms, safety factors are incorporated into the pacemaker. First, if the spontaneous atrial rate falls below the pacemaker's fixed rate, the pacemaker automatically converts to stimulate the ventricles at the preset fixed rate and ceases to function for that period of time as a P-wave sensor. Second, the maximum rate at which the pacemaker will fire is approximately 165 pulses per minute. When this rate is reached, a limiting circuit within the generator will induce a 2:1 block, halving the ventricular rate, and producing an actual rate of 82 to 83 pulses per minute. If the atrial rate continues to increase, the limiting circuit will not allow its actual output rate to exceed 165 pulses per minute; this is accomplished by producing proportionately higher blocks (3:1, 4:1, 5:1, etc). Activation of the limiting circuit can be recognized by the abrupt decrease in the output rate of the pacemaker in response to faster atrial rates.

A final safety feature is that stray magnetic impulses from the environment (EMI) cannot by themselves alter the programmed rate. Nevertheless, patients should be cautioned against coming close to EMI sources. Physicians should also exercise caution around these patients, especially with electrocauterization and diathermy.

The proliferation of pacemakers with varying sensing and pacing modes led to much confusion in terminology. In attempts to clarify matters, the Inter-Society Commission for Heart Disease Resources proposed a nomenclature code to identify the mode of operation of the pulse generator. This code consists of three letters, which indicate the chamber paced, the chamber sensed, and the mode of response, in that order. The letters used to identify the chambers are A for atrium, V for ventricles, and O for both chambers. The mode of response is identified by I for inhibited, T for

*Dr. P.J. Bower

triggered; O is used when neither is applicable, such as in asynchronous or fixed-rate pacemakers. In regard to the pacemaker implanted in the patient presented here, the following apply: 1) the chamber paced is the ventricle-V; 2) the chamber sensed is the atrium-A; 3) the generator is discharged by the sensed atrial signal-T. Thus, the proper nomenclature is VAT.

## SELECTED READINGS

Fruman S: The present status of cardiac pacing. *Surg Gynecol Obstet* 143:645, 1976.

Lown B, Kosowsky BD: Artificial pacemakers. *N Engl J Med* 283:907, 1970.

Parsonnet V, et al: Implantable cardiac pacemakers: status report and resource guideline. *Circulation* 50:A-21, 1974.

Smyth NPD: Cardiac pacing. *Ann Thorac Surg* 27:270, 1979.

Smyth NPD, et al: The pacemaker patient and the electromagnetic environment. *JAMA* 227:1412, 1974.

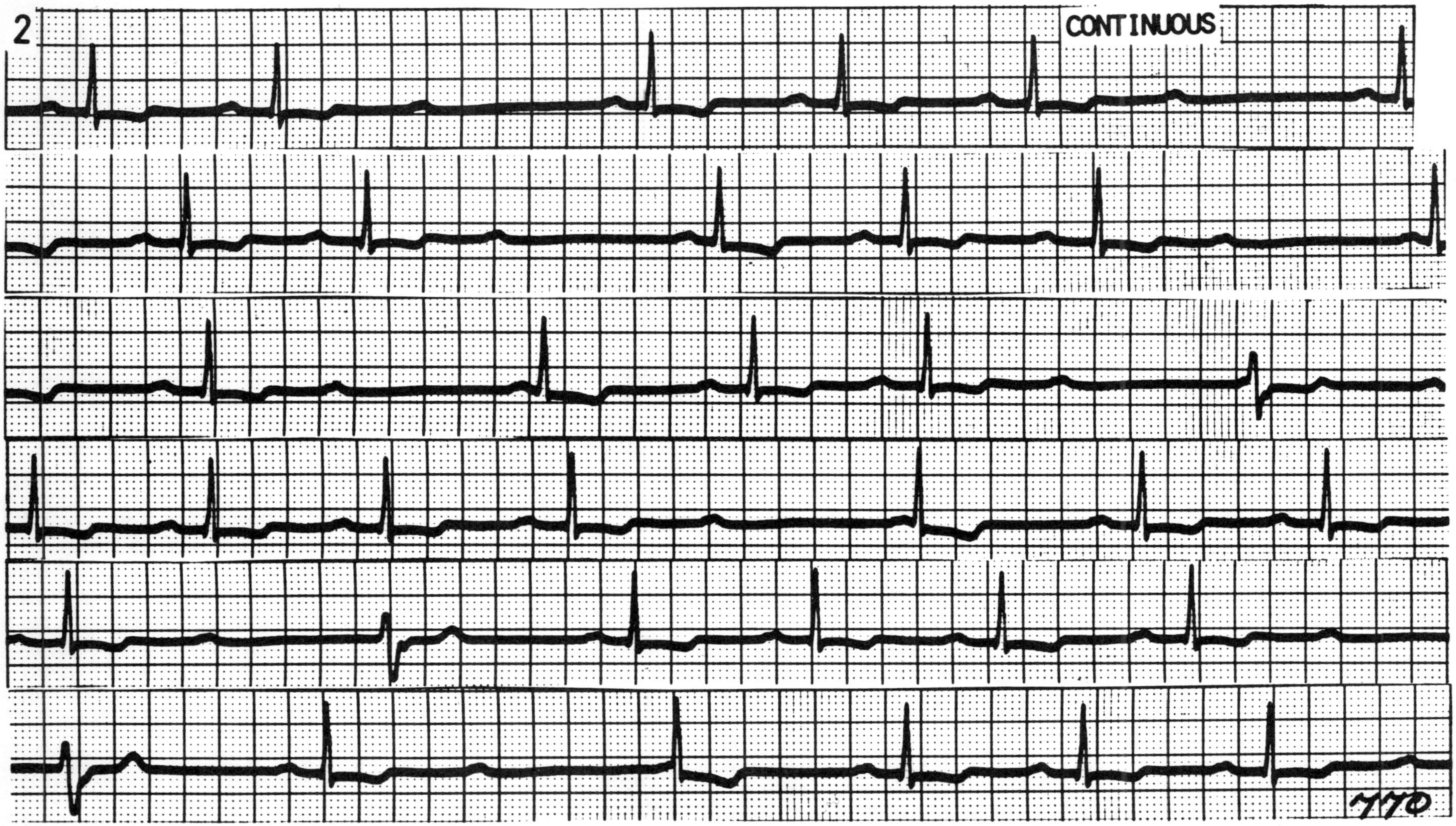


**Figure 3** This tracing was taken on a 72-year-old man found to have an ''irregular pulse,'' with a previous diagnosis of ''alcoholic cardiomyopathy.'' He was on no medications.

# NUMBER 3 *Eeny, Meeny, Miny,...Mobitz* Jorge I. Martinez-Lopez

## ELUCIDATION

**Diagnosis**—*Atypical Mobitz type I AV block*

The supraventricular impulse originates in the sinus node, and the variability in the P-P intervals is consistent with sinus arrhythmia. Atrial pathology can be suspected in view of the wide, notched P waves. Normal intraventricular conduction is present, ie, narrow QRS complexes.

Prominent features of the rhythm strips are: 1) progressive prolongation of the P-R intervals; 2) intermittent pauses alternating with clusters of ventricular complexes (group-beating); and, 3) escape beats.

A number of phenomena in the tracing makes it different from the classical Mobitz type I AV block (Wenckebach). In most instances, the P-R interval of the first conducted sinus beat is prolonged (first-degree AV block) and fixed. On occasion, however, the first conducted P waves "moves in" closer to (4th and 8th P waves in 2nd row, 3rd P wave in 3rd row; 5th P wave in 4th row), or is "lost" in (3rd QRS complex in bottom row) the QRS complex. From this, it can be inferred that the mechanisms involved are the fortuitous occurrence of a nonconducted sinus beat and a junctional escape beat.

Ventricular escape beats are also present (5th QRS complex in 3rd row, 2nd QRS in 4th row, 1st QRS in bottom row). They prolong the pause which follows the blocked sinus beat by creating an area of refractoriness at the nodal-His through concealed retrograde condition. In effect, therefore, two sinus beats are blocked; one by the decremental conduction of the Wenckebach cycle, and the second by concealed retrograde penetration of the junctional area by the escape beat.

## DISCUSSION

Traditionally, second-degree AV block (Mobitz block) is classified into two types, based upon the behavior of the P-R intervals before the blocked atrial beat. Second-degree block characterized by progressive prolongation of the P-R intervals is termed *Mobitz type I AV block* (Wenckebach phenomenon, Wenckebach periodicity); *in Mobitz type II AV block,* the P-R intervals are fixed.

His bundle electrocardiography and other intracavitary recordings have greatly enhanced our understanding of patterns of abnormal AV conduction. Accordingly, not only have diagnostic criteria come under closer scrutiny, but so have the concepts of management and prognosis. Currently, it is generally agreed that both type I and II block may occur with either functional or structural abnormality of the conduction system, and both may reflect either nodal or infranodal conduction disturbance. The prognosis of second-degree AV block appears to be dependent upon the site of the block. Thus, block proximal to the His bundle is usually benign and distal block usually malignant. The discussion which follows is limited exclusively to Mobitz type I AV block.

Mobitz type I AV block is one of the most common electrophysiologic phenomena in the human heart. During sinus rhythm, the *classical* form exhibits the following features.

1. Progressive prolongation of the *P-R intervals* is present.
2. Successive *P-R increments* progressively diminish.
3. The ventricular rate accelerates and is reflected in progressive diminution of the R-R interval.
4. The pause resulting from the blocked sinus impulses is equal to the sum of the increments subtracted from twice the P-P interval.
5. The R-R interval following the pause is *always* longer than the R-R interval preceding the pause.

Normal sinus rhythm, however, *is not* essential to the diagnosis of Mobitz type I AV block. Wenckebach periodicity may be recognized in association with paroxysmal atrial tachycardia, atrial flutter, junctional tachycardia, and junctional escape rhythm. In any of these, a constant ratio of supraventricular to conducted impulses in a given sequence leads to group-beating. With varying conduction ratios, a completely irregular ventricular rhythm results.

While the *classical* form of Mobitz type I AV block is easily recognized by conventional electrocardiography, *variants* are not infrequent and may be the source of confusion, posing problems in interpretation. Some of these are briefly discussed below.

In most instances of Wenckebach periodicity, QRS complexes are normal in duration. Abnormally wide ventricular complexes occur in the presence of established bundle branch block or when refractory periods of the bundle branches are unequal (phasic aberrant conduction).

Not all blocked atrial beats are followed by a normally conducted P wave. The blocked impulse may be followed by either a junctional or ventricular escape beat and, depending upon the location of the escape beat in the sequence, it may be coincidental with, or mask the conduction of, the first beat of the next Wenckebach sequence. Moreover, it must be recognized that the P wave (or F wave, in atrial flutter) immediately preceding a QRS complex does not necessarily represent the conducted supraventricular impulse. Close examination of long rhythm strips permits this distinction.

The Wenckebach sequence may be followed by two or more consecutively blocked supraventricular impulses, particularly in the presence of the so-called *alternating Wenckebach periodicity,* and may be mistaken for high grade AV block.

In the presence of marked sinus arrhythmia or long series of conducted beats before the dropped beat, the P-R intervals may be variable and appear haphazard. Also, long sequences of Wenckebach periodicity may exhibit several *constant* P-R intervals before the dropped beat, leading to the erroneous diagnosis of Mobitz type II AV block.

In exceptional cases, the Wenckebach sequence *is not* terminated by a blocked atrial beat. Instead, the sequence ends with an atrial "echo" beat or with a reciprocating tachycardia. In others, concealed retrograde conduction of an atrial "echo" beat may prevent the progressive diminution of R-R intervals.

A final word of caution. Fixed 2:1 AV block should not be classified as type II block, regardless of the duration of QRS complexes, for it may represent a 2:1 Wenckebach sequence. Long rhythm strips may assist in resolving the issue if other conduction ratios (3:2, 4:3, etc) appear during the recording.

## SELECTED READINGS

Amat y Leon F, et al: Alternating Wenckebach periodicity: a common electrophysiologic response. *Am J Cardiol* 36:757–764, 1975.

Barold SS, et al: Second degree atrioventricular block. A matter of definition. *Am J Cardiol* 33:311–314, 1974.

Dreifus LS, et al: Atrioventricular block. *Am J Cardiol* 28:371–380, 1971.

El-Sherif N, et al: Pathophysiology of second degree atrioventricular block: a unified hypothesis. *Am J Cardiol* 35:421–424, 1975.

Langendorf R, et al: Observations on second degree atrioventricular block, including new criteria for the differential diagnosis between type I and type II block. *Am J Cardiol* 29:111–119, 1972.

## NUMBER 4 *Playing with Blocks* Jorge I. Martinez-Lopez

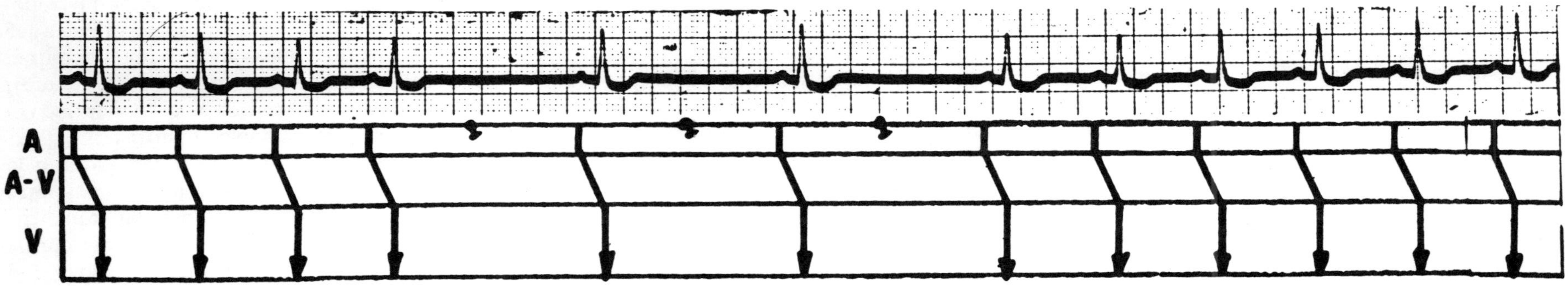


**Figure 4** This tracing is of a 65-year-old man complaining of intermittent dizziness. He was on no medications.

**NUMBER 4** *Playing with Blocks* Jorge I. Martinez-Lopez

## ELUCIDATION

**Diagnosis**—*Second degree SA block*

The basic mechanism is sinus in nature. The P-R and QRS intervals are normal in duration.

The prominent feature of the tracing is the abrupt pause which follows the fourth QRS complex. This first pause is followed by two more pauses of equal duration to the first one before resumption of the faster sinus rate.

Careful measurement of the P-P intervals of the faster rate preceding the pauses and "marching" them through, shows that the P-P intervals of the pauses accommodate two basic sinus cycles. Accordingly, a diagnosis of intermittent second degree (2:1) SA block can be established.

## DISCUSSION

The sinoatrial node (SAN) is the normal pacemaker for the heart. Impulse formation within the SAN is an inherent property of this structure. Its rate of firing is influenced—accelerated or reduced—by a variety of external or internal factors alone or in combination.

For the atria to be depolarized as a prelude to contraction, the electrical activity must exist from the SAN, cross an anatomical barrier—the perinodal buffer zone—,and spread centrifugally and perhaps down the internodal and interatrial tracts to the atrial musculature. Consequently, SAN dysfunction can be the result of disturbances in impulse formation, impulse conduction, or both.

Disturbances in impulse conduction analogous to those occurring in the AV node can occur in the SAN, presumably at the perinodal buffer zone *(exit block),* and are referred to as *sinoatrial block* (SAB). In SAB, the SAN continues to discharge regularly but the impulses are either delayed on their way out of the node or are blocked intermittently or permanently.

Sinoatrial block has been reported to occur in clinically normal and abnormal hearts under the influence of toxic, chemical, and psychological factors. It has also been observed during swallowing and micturition in normal persons. Systemic arterial hypertension, and rheumatic and coronary artery disease are the most frequent disorders associated with SAB. Even in the presence of established cardiac disease, remember that SAB *may not always* have a structural basis, for it may last a short period of time or even several years and then disappear spontaneously. Atropine in large doses and exercise can temporarily abolish the arrhythmia.

Diagnosis of all cases *is not* always possible from the surface ECG. *First-degree* SAB occurs when the sinus impulses are delayed in being conducted into the atrial musculature. Since the formation of the sinus impulse *is not* reflected on the ECG, this type of block cannot be recognized clinically. In *third-degree* (complete) SAB, none of the sinus impulses emerge and, failing to reach the atria, result in absence of P waves. Since the atria and ventricles are distal to the site of block, escape rhythms become the dominant pacemakers of the heart. Consequently, this type of block cannot be distinguished from failure of impulse formation (sinus arrest), atrial standstill, and sinoventricular conduction and rhythm.

Second-degree SAB is recognizable from the surface ECG. Two types, analogous to Mobitz I and II AV block, are observed; ie, *with* and *without* Wenckebach phenomena. The presence of a pause involving a complete cardiac cycle should prompt the interpreter to consider SAB, but it may also be the result of a long intermission occurring in sinus arrhythmia, or of temporary failure of impulse formation in the SAN.

The presence of sinus Wenckebach periods can be inferred by observation and calculation of the rhythmic sequences involving the P-P intervals. The conduction interval from the SAN to the atrial musculature (S-A interval) progressively increases until conduction fails completely and a sinus impulse is "dropped." From this concept, the following criteria evolve for the electrocardiographic recognition of Wenckebach periods in SAB:

1. There is a gradual shortening of the P-P interval preceding the pause. The reason is that, although the S-A interval becomes progressively longer, the increment by which it increases becomes progressively smaller. Hence, P-P interval shortens; ie, the atrial rate accelerates before the "dropped" sinus impulse.

2. The P-P interval *including* the blocked sinus impulse is shorter than twice the distance of the P-P interval preceding it. This holds true if only one impulse is blocked. When two or

more are suspected to be blocked, calculation of the basic sinus cycle (using Schamroth's formulae) is vitally important.

3. The P-P interval *after* the blocked sinus impulse is longer than that preceding the pause.

Wenckebach sequences in SAB must be differentiated from sinus arrhythmia and from sinus extrasystoles. Bigeminal rhythm, resulting from 3:2 SAB, mimics atrial premature stimuli.

Sinoatrial block analogous to Mobitz II AV block is also recognizable on the surface electrocardiogram. In this instance, there is a failure of conduction of one or alternating sinus impulses. When the sinus impulse is blocked, a complete P-QRS-T cycle is "dropped." The regular discharge of the SAN during the pause can be inferred by demonstrating that the long pause is a multiple of the basic sinus cycle. Regular 2:1 SAB, however, may be impossible to differentiate from chronic sinus bradycardia clinically or by ECG.

Symptoms may be totally absent. When present, symptoms do not reflect the SAN dysfunction but rather an abnormality of the escape function of subsidiary pacemakers. Not uncommonly, SAB is also complicated by supraventricular arrhythmias and AV conduction disturbances. Such patients may experience cerebral ischemia with syncope, episodes of rapid palpitations, or both.

Management is dependent upon the cause of SAB. Removal of toxic, chemical, and psychological factors may abolish the arrythmia. In the remainder, drug therapy is ineffective, and permanent pacemaking is required.

## SELECTED READINGS

Myerburg RJ, El-Sherif N: Electrocardiographic diagnosis of sinus rhythmic variations and sinoatrial block, in *Advances in Electrocardiography*. New York, Grune & Stratton Inc, 1976, pp 59–70.

Obel IWP, Cohen E, Miller RNS: Chronic symptomatic sinoatrial block. *Chest* 65:397–402, 1974.

Schamroth L, Dove E: The Wenckebach phenomenon in sino-atrial block. *Br Heart J* 28:350–358, 1966.

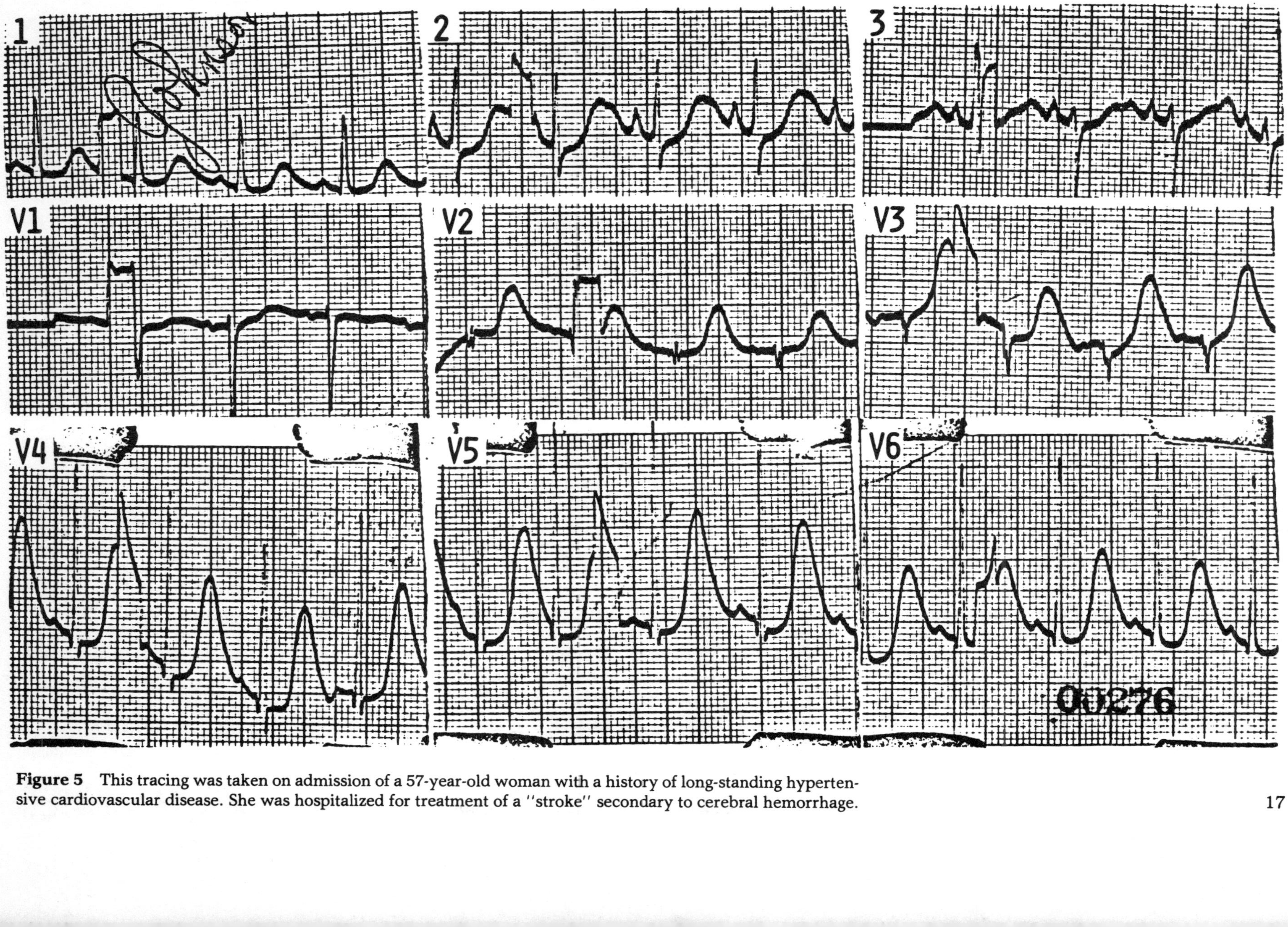


**Figure 5** This tracing was taken on admission of a 57-year-old woman with a history of long-standing hypertensive cardiovascular disease. She was hospitalized for treatment of a "stroke" secondary to cerebral hemorrhage.

## NUMBER 5 *No Stroke of Luck* Jorge I. Martinez-Lopez

### ELUCIDATION

In the analysis of the electrocardiogram there is normal sinus rhythm. The P waves are prominent and peaked in leads 2 and 3. Nonspecific sagging ST segments are present. The amplitude of the QRS complexes in the lateral precordial leads is compatible with left ventricular hypertrophy. The Q-T interval is prolonged. The T waves are upright but are extremely wide and tall.

### DISCUSSION

Certain electrocardiographic abnormalities have been observed in patients with central nervous system disease in the absence of demonstrable heart disease and coexisting electrolyte disturbances. Cerebral disorders include intracranial hemorrhage, cerebrovascular accidents, and tumors of the central nervous system. Changes have also been noted postoperatively in patients operated on for cerebral disorders.

It appears that cerebral disorders can produce disturbances in depolarization and repolarization of the myocardium, as well as cardiac arrhythmias. The ECG changes include the following: a) prominent and peaked P waves; b) shortened P-R interval; c) abnormal Q waves; d) prolongation, depression, or elevation of the ST segment; e) extremely wide and prominent T waves, either tall and upright or deeply inverted; f) Q-T prolongation; and g) prominent U waves. Disturbances of impulse conduction are infrequently seen.

The specter of life-threatening cardiac arrhythmias is potentially present. This has led to the suggestion that these patients should be treated in coronary care units where special facilities are available for continuous monitoring of the ECG and for managing serious arrhythmias. Circulatory arrest secondary to ventricular fibrillation is not an infrequent cause of death.

What do the ECG abnormalities represent? The exact relationship of the cerebral insult to the ECG changes is not entirely clear. It is probable that such cerebral abnormalities must involve, among other areas, the hypothalamic area, either extrinsically or intrinsically. Electrical stimulation of specialized areas in the brain of experimental animals can produce ECG patterns of the WPW syndrome as well as AV dissociation. ECG changes have also been noted shortly after injection of paraffin into the carotid artery of experimental animals. Other studies have revealed different innervation of the anterior and posterior halves of the ventricles: the right stellate ganglion supplying the anterior half; the left, the posterior half. These suggest that ECG abnormalities may be related to nonhomogeneity in refractory periods of the ventricles brought about by unilateral alteration in sympathetic tone.

Histologic changes in the myocardium have been seen in a number of patients dying from central nervous disease, either with or without ECG changes. These include subendocardial hemorrhage, focal areas of myocytolysis, and ultrastructural changes in the myocardium. There is some evidence to suggest that the development of such lesions may also be mediated by alterations in the autonomic nervous system. Other investigators have found no such myocardial lesions. Hence, the relationship of the myocardial to the ECG changes remains controversial.

Finally, ECG abnormalities also have been noted in brain death (coma depassé). These are probably determined by the dual influence of the depressant effect of the associated hypothermia and the stimulating action of the sympathetic nervous system.

### SELECTED READINGS


Abildskov JA, Millar K, Burgess MJ, et al: The electrocardiogram and the central nervous system. *Prog Cardiovasc Dis* 13:210, 1970.

Hunt D, Gore I: Myocardial lesions following experimental intracranial hemorrhage: prevention with propranolol. *Am Heart J* 83:232, 1972.

Mauck HP Jr, Hockman CH: Central nervous system mechanisms mediating cardiac rate and rhythm. *Am Heart J* 74:96, 1967.

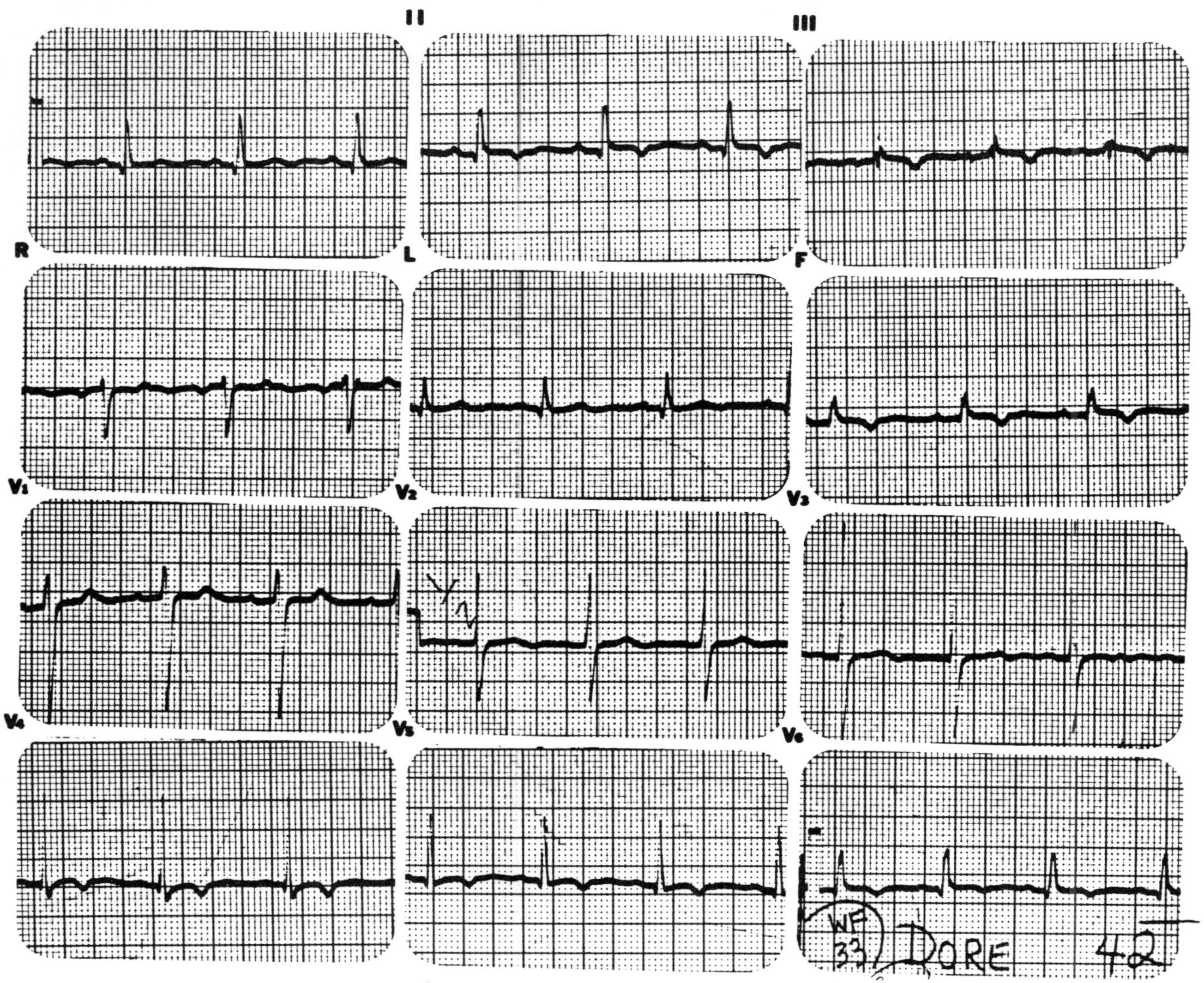


**Figure 6** This tracing is of a 32-year-old woman with a one-month history of intermittent, nonexertional precordial pain. The pain did not radiate. Six months previously, a routine physical examination first disclosed an apical systolic murmur. At the time the electrocardiogram was recorded, she was on no medications.

# NUMBER 6 *Coronary Artery Disease Mimic* Jorge I. Martinez-Lopez

## ELUCIDATION

An electrocardiograph (ECG) analysis shows a sinus rhythm. The P-R, QRS and Q-T intervals and the electrical axis are all within normal limits.

The major abnormal feature is the inversion of T waves in leads II, III, AVF, and $V_4$ through $V_6$, which suggest ischemia of the inferolateral wall of the left ventricle. Prominent U waves are also noted in most leads.

## DISCUSSION

The tracing is that of a patient with *the mitral valve prolapse-click syndrome.*

Physical examination revealed the presence of a midsystolic click, followed by a late systolic murmur at the apex. Left ventricular angiography demonstrated systolic prolapse of the posterior leaflet of the mitral valve into the left atrium with mitral regurgitation, and an area of abnormal contractility on the inferior wall.

The syndrome occurs predominantly in women, and it may be familial or congenital. Over half of the patients with this condition experience atypical precordial pain, dyspnea, palpitations, and/or lightheadedness.

The clinical features of the syndrome make the diagnosis at the bedside relatively easy, and include either a midsystolic click, a late systolic murmur, or both. Once the diagnosis is suspected, it can be readily confirmed by noninvasive procedures, such as echocardiography and apexcardiography, and also by left ventriculoangiography. Although the prognosis is usually benign, sudden death and subacute bacterial endocarditis of the mitral valve have been reported.

Electrocardiographic abnormalities are common. Inversion of the T waves in leads II, III, and AVF is probably the most common variation, but abnormal T waves may be observed in other leads, apparently depending on which mitral leaflet prolapses and whether one or both leaflets prolapse. In patients with the syndrome who have a normal resting electrocardiogram, T wave abnormalities may be evoked by inhalation of amyl nitrite.

The cause of the T wave inversion remains unknown, although a number of mechanisms have been postulated. Selective coronary arteriography is usually entirely normal in these patients, making it clear that obstructive lesions of the major coronary trunks are not responsible for the electrocardiographic changes.

Unusually large U waves have also been noted and have been thought to represent delayed repolarization of papillary muscles and related structures.

Arrhythmias may occur at rest in some cases, while in others stress testing can evoke cardiac irritability not present at rest. More commonly, there are premature ventricular contractions, either unifocal or multifocal, which presumably may be forerunners of more serious or lethal arrhythmias. Other electrocardiographic abnormalities noted include supraventricular arrhythmias, "infarction" QRS patterns, and Q-T prolongation.

## SELECTED READINGS


Jeresaty RM: Mitral valve prolapse-click syndrome. *Prog Cardiovasc Dis* 15:623–652, 1973.

Lobstein HP, Horwitz LD, Curry GC, et al: Electrocardiographic abnormalities and coronary arteriograms in the mitral click-murmur syndrome. *N Engl J Med* 289:127–131, 1973.

Pocock WA, Barlow JB: Etiology and electrocardiographic features of the billowing posterior mitral leaflet syndrome. *Am J Med* 51:731–739, 1971.

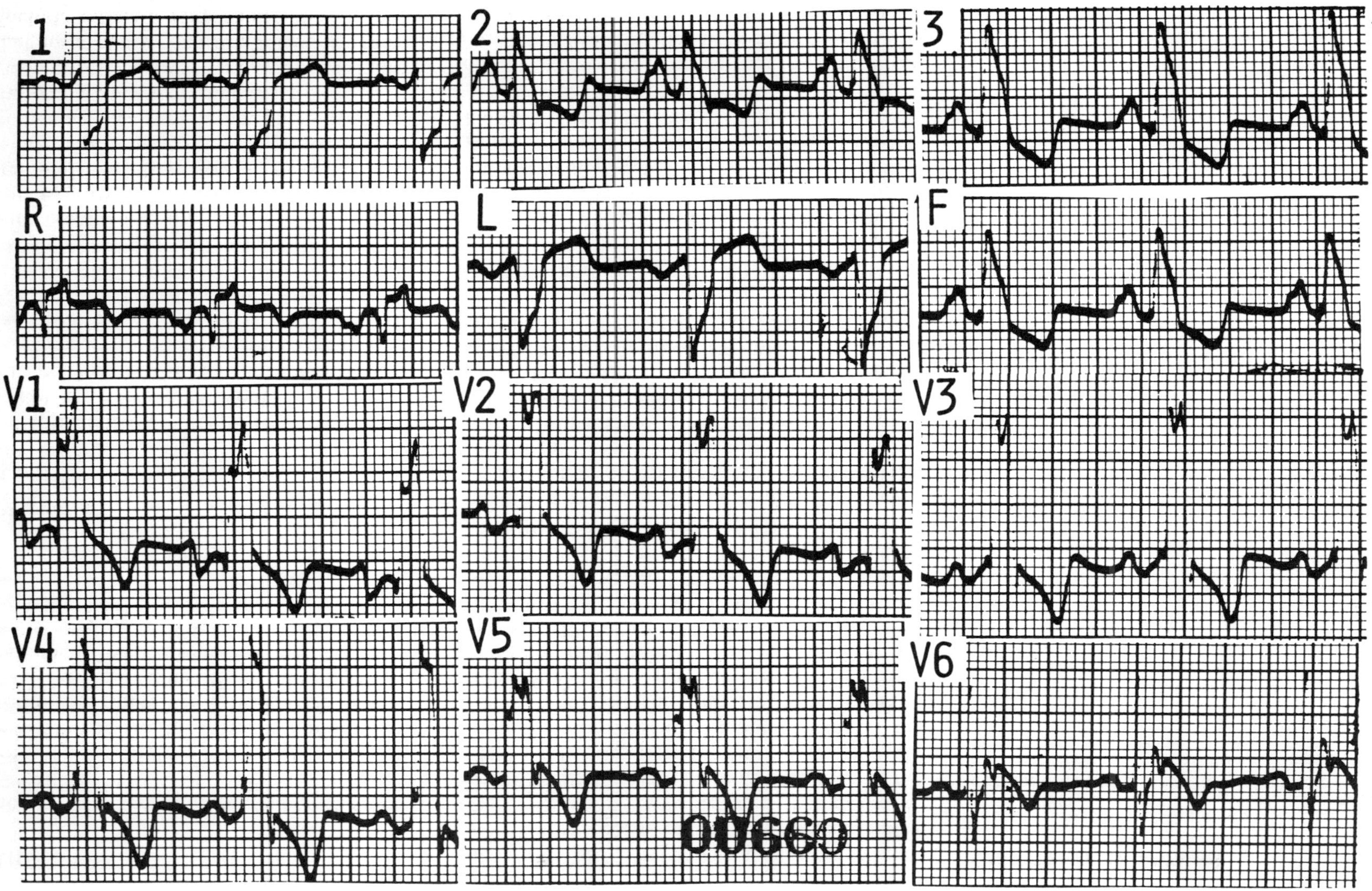


**Figure 7** This tracing was taken on a 17-year-old male several days after cardiac surgery for congenital cyanotic heart disease.

# NUMBER 7 *Iatrogenic Block—Central or Peripheral?* Jorge I. Martinez-Lopez

## ELUCIDATION

**Diagnosis**—*Complete right bundle branch block*

Normal sinus rhythm is present. The electrical axis in the frontal plane is abnormally deviated to the right. The P waves are broad and notched, indicating atrial pathology. A complete right bundle branch block (CRBBB) pattern is seen in the precordial leads. The ST segments and T waves show secondary changes.

## DISCUSSION

The appearance of CRBBB following right ventriculotomy has been attributed to surgical injury to portions of the right intraventricular system. This electrocardiographic complication has been the focus of recent interest and a source of controversy. Much of the controversy revolves around the precise mechanism, clinical significance, and prognosis of the iatrogenic conduction abnormality.

With regard to the mechanism by which CRBBB develops following right ventriculotomy, recent reports implicate two sites where injury can occur: centrally and peripherally, alone or in combination.

Earlier studies in patients undergoing right ventriculotomy strongly indicated that CRBBB was primarily or solely related to the ventricular incision. It was noted that in some instances CRBBB occurred immediately following the right ventricular incision *and prior* to correction of the cardiac anomaly. Other evidence also suggested that development of RBBB in those patients was likely to be related to the direction (vertical *vs* transverse), location, and total length of the incision on the free wall of the right ventricle. These conclusions were subsequently challenged because a relatively large number of patients *do not* develop CRBBB after a right ventriculotomy. Presently, the general consensus is that, in some patients, ventriculotomy-induced CRBBB is the result of disruption of a *peripheral* branch or branches of the right bundle branch or its arborization (peripheral right ventricular delay).

In another group of patients, postoperative CRBBB may result from a more *central* lesion (true RBBB) related to surgical trauma, injury or hemorrhage to the main right bundle.

A last group may be one in whom ventriculotomy-induced CRBBB is due to a combination of *peripheral* and *central* lesions.

Unfortunately, current electrocardiographic criteria do not provide a means of differentiating between the three groups. Okoroma et al, however, have expressed hope that analysis of the Frank vectorcardiogram will make it possible to differentiate central from peripheral injury by the appearance of the initial vectorcardiographic forces.

The prognostic significance of ventriculotomy-induced CRBBB has not been clarified yet. Claims have been made that it is associated with increased incidence of late complete heart block and sudden death, but other reports accord it a benign prognosis.

## SELECTED READINGS


Krongrad E, Hefler SE, Bowman FO Jr, et al: Further observations on the etiology of right bundle branch block pattern following right ventriculotomy. *Circulation* 50:1105, 1974.

Okoroma EO, Guller B, Maloney JD, et al: Etiology of right bundle branch block pattern after surgical closure of ventricular septal defects. *Am Heart J* 90:14, 1975.

Steeg CN, Krongrad E, Davachi F, et al: Postoperative left anterior hemiblock and right bundle branch block following repair of tetralogy of Fallot. *Circulation* 51:1026, 1975.

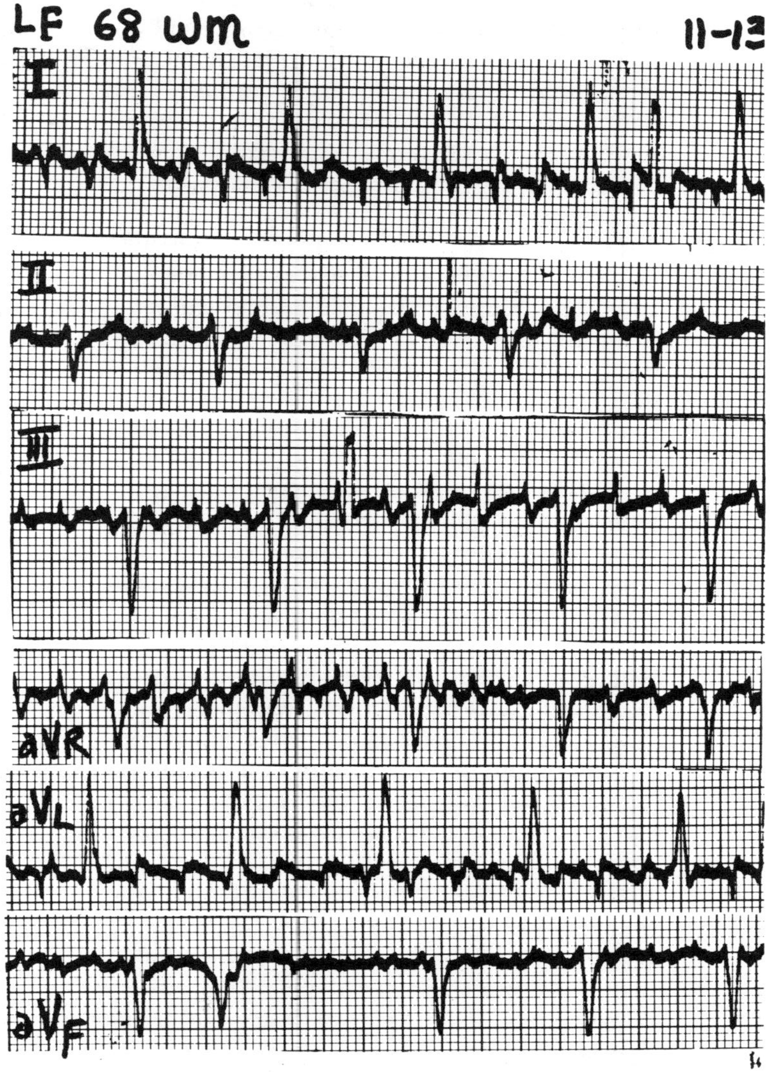


**Figure 8** The tracing was taken in a 56-year-cld man, a prospective candidate for a drug study, as part of his preliminary assessment before the experimental drug was started. There was no known history of heart disease, and he was on no medications.

# NUMBER 8 *Trick or Treat?* Jorge I. Martinez-Lopez

## ELUCIDATION

**Diagnosis**—*Pseudo-atrial flutter*

The ventricular rate is regular, at 84 per minute. The QRS complexes are narrow, indicating normal intraventricular conduction of supraventricular impulses. Abnormal left axis deviation is present. The second beat in lead $aV_F$ represents a ventricular premature beat.

The prominent feature in the tracing, however, is the presence of biphasic "waves" between adjacent QRS complexes occurring regularly, at a rapid rate (about 260 per minute), and suggesting atrial flutter with physiologic AV block. At times, these oscillations have a "spiked" configuration. These "waves" are in reality produced by parkinsonian tremor, and successfully conceal normal P waves. The patient was in normal sinus rhythm.

## DISCUSSION

Artifacts have been documented repeatedly in the 12-lead resting electrocardiogram, with use of bipolar chest leads in coronary care units, and in portable electrocardiographic monitoring. Artifactual distortions in the ECG may mimic arrhythmias (pseudoarrhythmias) or create alterations in atrial and/or ventricular complexes, ST segments, and T waves. Such changes may lead to errors in interpretation and therapy when they go unrecognized.

Two main sources of artifacts are *electrical* and *mechanical*. The latter is most frequently the result of *somatic (bodily) tremor*. Numerous conditions may be associated with somatic tremor, among which are: tension caused by fear and apprehension, shaking, parkinsonism, hyperthyroidism, clonic contractions of at least one extremity in cerebral disease, and hiccups. In a patient being monitored with a bipolar chest lead, use of an electric razor to shave produced artifacts simulating atrial flutter in the monitor scope and in the rhythm strip (WP Nelson, personal communication).

Recognition of such artifacts may be difficult and at times almost impossible. A high index of suspicion on the part of the interpreter is a necessary ingredient. Cheng and Efpraxiades have proposed the use of one or more of the following criteria to establish the correct diagnosis of "pseudoatrial flutter": a) baseline oscillations not very regular in rhythm; b) deflections not even in size and shape, sharp at times and blunt at other times; c) waxing and waning of amplitude and frequency; d) usually intermittent in occurrence; e) regular ventricular rate unaffected by the onset of "pseudoatrial flutter"; f) no constant relationship between the last oscillation and the next ventricular complex; g) sinus P waves may be identified in some leads; h) localization of "pseudoatrial flutter" to several leads only; i) "pseudoatrial flutter" waves should be traceable to a particular group of skeletal muscles responsible for the tremors which are usually grossly visible.

Obviously, difficulty with artifacts should be overcome *before they occur*—if possible—through proper technique. Every effort should be made to obtain a recording of high quality and fidelity. But, on occasion, even with the best of care, distortions will pop up to haunt both the technician and the interpreter. If proper precautions do not minimize or eliminate artifacts, the person recording the tracing bears the responsibility of alerting the interpreter.

In patients with parkinsonism, one may obviate difficulties encountered with the tremor by reattaching the bipolar arm lead wires at the shoulders, or the leg connections as high as possible. If this maneuver has no effect on the tremor artifact and the presence of an arrhythmia remains in question, the technician should "automatically" record a rhythm strip using either the Golub or the Lewis lead.

Trick or treat? *Trick!*

## SELECTED READINGS

Cheng TO, Efpraxiades J: Pseudo-atrial flutter. *Chest* 57:290–292, 1970.

## NUMBER 9 *Lung Gone* Jorge I. Martinez-Lopez

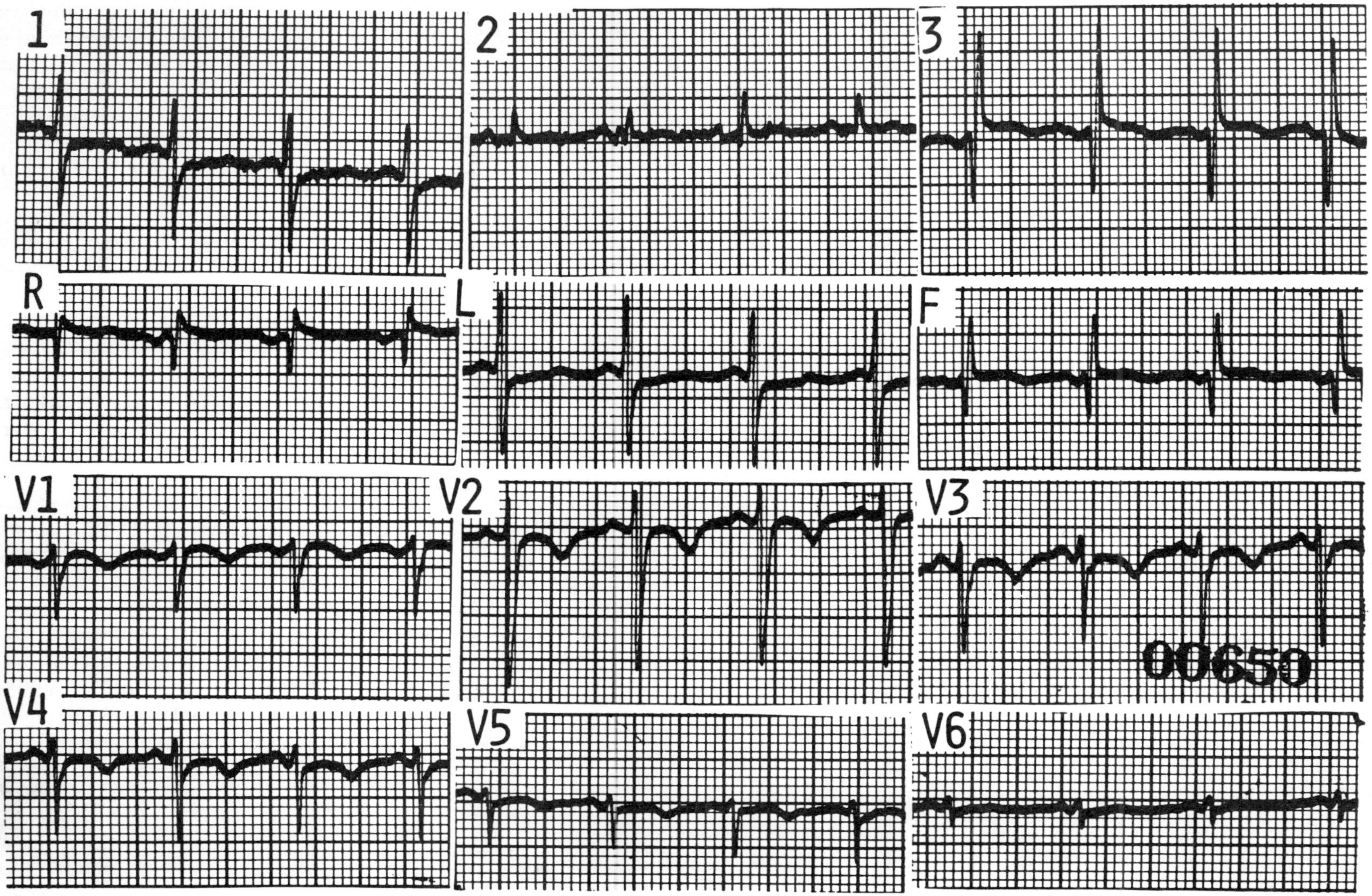


**Figure 9** The tracing was taken in a 34-year-old woman, with a long-standing history of wheezing. Twenty-one years earlier she had undergone lung surgery. Scoliosis of the thoracic spine with concavity to the right was present. She was on no medications.

# NUMBER 9 *Lung Gone* Jorge I. Martinez-Lopez

## ELUCIDATION

There is sinus tachycardia with normal PR, QRS, and QT intervals, and right axis deviation. Nonspecific ST-segment and T-wave changes are present in all of the leads. Poor R-wave progression and gradual reduction in the amplitude of the QRS complexes are noted from the right to the left precordial leads.

These most unusual changes are consistent with marked cardiac rotation following pneumonectomy. In this patient, the left lung was removed 21 years earlier because of bronchiectasis. No cardiac disease or evidence of myocardial damage was present then or subsequently.

## DISCUSSION

Pulmonary operations may be complicated by early or late abnormalities in cardiac hemodynamics and/or the electrocardiogram. Transient *cardiac arrhythmias* are observed in approximately 30% of patients during the first five days after surgery. Atrial fibrillation is the most common, usually yielding rapidly to intravenous administration of digitalis. Other acute changes include deviations in the electrical axis, ST-segment and T-wave changes, myocardial infarction, and conduction abnormalities.

Removal of one lung usually results in marked shift of the heart into the ipsilateral hemithorax, unless the mediastinum is fixed by disease. Rotatory displacement generally accompanies the shift in location.

*Positional* and *rotatory changes* characterize the late postpneumonectomy electrocardiographic tracings. When the heart is displaced to the right after right pneumonectomy, the heart rotates counterclockwise, but not to an extreme degree. The 12-lead electrocardiogram shows deep Q waves in leads I, II, $V_{5\text{-}6}$. Upright T waves are usually present, unless underlying cardiac disease or other factors affecting its polarity are present. The transition complexes are shifted rightward in the precordial leads; hence tall R waves are recorded in the right chest leads. These features are thus related to dextroposition and must be differentiated from dextrocardia and dextroversion. Caution should also be taken in making a diagnosis of right ventricular hypertrophy without taking additional leads to the right.

In contrast, left pneumonectomy results in right axis deviation and clockwise rotation of the heart along its longitudinal axis, both attributable to positional changes of the heart in the hemithorax. In addition, approximately 50% of these patients show a pattern of incomplete right bundle branch block in $V_1$. "P pulmonale" is not a common feature.

Lobectomies and lesser lung resections generally show little or no shift in cardiac position; hence no changes are recorded in the electrocardiogram.

## SELECTED READINGS


Calleja HB: Diagnostic value of electrocardiographic changes in pneumonectomies. *Cardiologia* 49:228–238, 1966.

Calleja HB, Asuncion RG: The electrocardiogram after lung resection in children. *Dis Chest* 50:456–463, 1966.

Stougard J: Cardiac arrhythmias following pneumonectomy. *Thorax* 24:568–572, 1969.

# NUMBER 10 *Out on a Limb* Jorge I. Martinez-Lopez

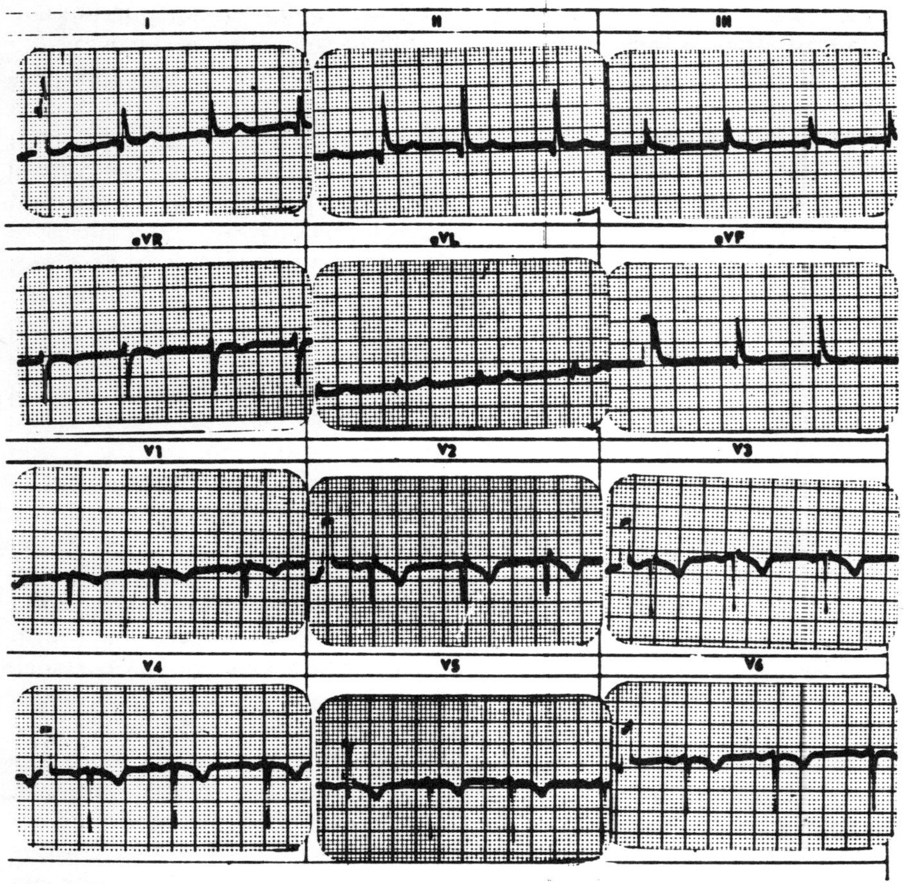


Figure 10-1

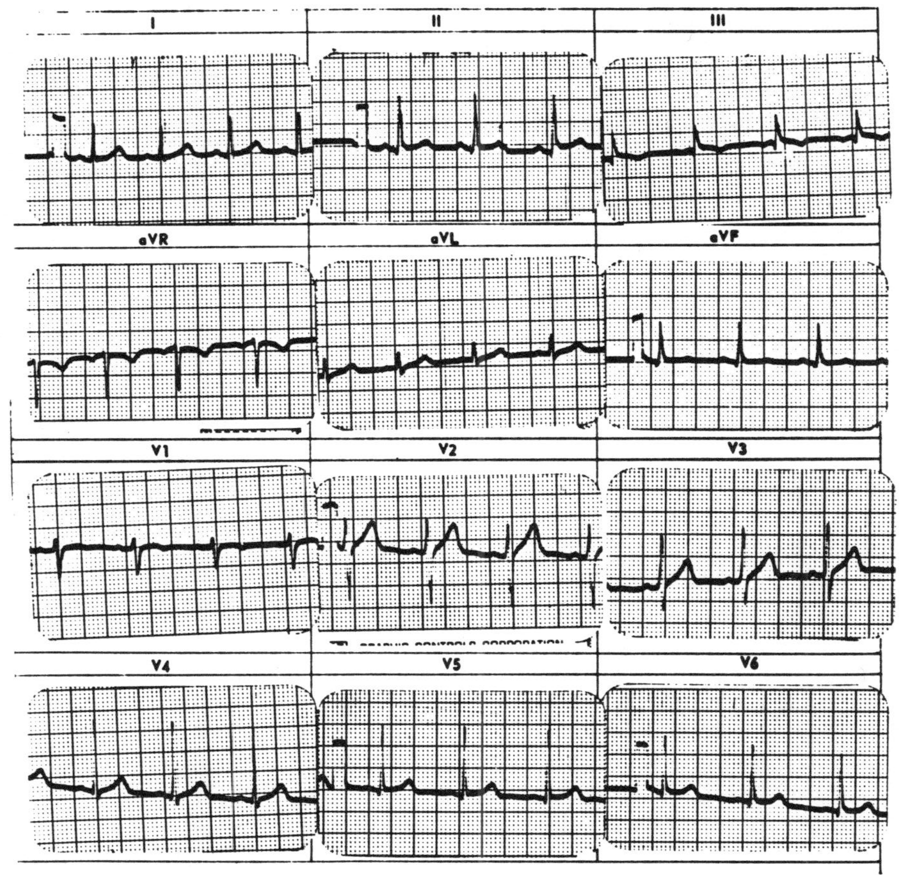


Figure 10-2

**Figure 10** The 12-lead resting tracing (Figure 10-1) is of a 25-year-old male executive, who requested a "routine" electrocardiogram because of recent onset of atypical anterior chest pain. He was on no medications. Figure 10-2 shows normal tracing with leads properly placed.

# NUMBER 10 *Out on a Limb* Jorge I. Martinez-Lopez

## ELUCIDATION

**Diagnosis**—*Improper electrode placement*

Normal sinus rhythm is present. The PR, QRS, and QT intervals are within normal limits.

The prominent features of the tracing are seen in the precordial leads. First, all the leads look very similar and bear a resemblance to AVR. Second, the normal progression of the R wave from right to left precordium never materializes. Instead, deep Q waves are noted from $V_1$ through $V_3$, and diminutive R waves from $V_4$ through $V_6$. Third, the T waves are deeply inverted over the entire precordium. Lastly, the P waves are also inverted and there are no significant changes in their morphology.

The "abnormal" appearance of the ECG raised serious questions. The tracing was recorded by a trainee—his first one—who, fortunately, had left the electrodes in place. When inspecting for electrode placement, it was found that the precordial lead wire (PLW) was attached to the right arm and the right-arm lead wire (RAW) was used as the "precordial" exploring electrode. The electrodes were then connected properly, and the second tracing (Figure 10-2) was normal.

## DISCUSSION

The conventional ECG utilizes leads which are *bipolar* (standard limb leads) and *unipolar* (precordial and augmented limb leads). Selection of the lead to be recorded is accomplished automatically by turning a switch without having to attach and detach the lead wires. This simplicity is a drawback because the electrocardiographic machine *does not* recognize errors introduced by improper placement of lead wires. Accordingly, polarity and configuration of P-QRS-T complexes may be altered and lead to erroneous interpretation of the tracing.

In order to understand the "abnormal" tracing presented (Figure 10-1), it is necessary to touch briefly upon certain facts. The basic arrangement of the *unipolar leads* calls for the limb electrodes to be connected to a central terminal, which becomes the negative pole at relative zero potential (indifferent electrode). In this manner only the positive pole explores the electrical field of the heart from the surface of the chest or from one of the limbs. For the augmented limb leads, however, the exploring limb lead is automatically disengaged from the central terminal by the switch and now compares the voltage across that lead with the average voltage across the two opposite limb electrodes.

In the case presented here, PLW was placed on the right arm and RAW was used to explore the six precordial locations. When the limb leads were recorded, RAW was already placed in the $V_1$ position; lead I now registered the difference in potential between the left arm and the location of RAW (now on the chest); and lead II, between the left leg and RAW. Similarly, with the switch turned to the AVR position, the voltage recorded from RAW was really from the $V_1$ location as the vantage point, and compared it with the average voltage across the remaining two limb electrodes. Accordingly, readings from these leads did not show any unusual alterations.

This was not the case with the precordial leads. When the switch was turned to the V position, PLW was still attached to the right arm, and the "viewing" area was from the right arm for all six precordial recordings. But, since RAW was used as the precordial "exploring" electrode and remained attached to the central terminal, the tracings obtained resembled those taken from the AVR position. The minor differences in configuration noted would be predictable since the relative zero of the central terminal would change each time the RAW was moved to a new precordial location.

The physician must be forever on the alert because errors such as this are common, and may not only lead to erroneous diagnosis but also to unnecessary treatment. Marriott has aptly termed them *"electrocardiographogenic suicide."*

## SELECTED READINGS


Dhingra RC, Wyndham C, Ehsani AA, et al: Left anterior hemiblock concealing diaphragmatic infarction and simulating anteroseptal infarction. *Chest* 67:713–715, 1975.

Horwitz S, Medrano GA: Left anterior hemiblock or inadvertent lead misplacement? *Chest* 69:449–450, 1976.

Marriott HJL: Electrocardiographogenic suicide and lesser crimes. *J Fla Med Assoc* 50:440, 1963.

# NUMBER 11 *See the U-turn?* Jorge I. Martinez-Lopez

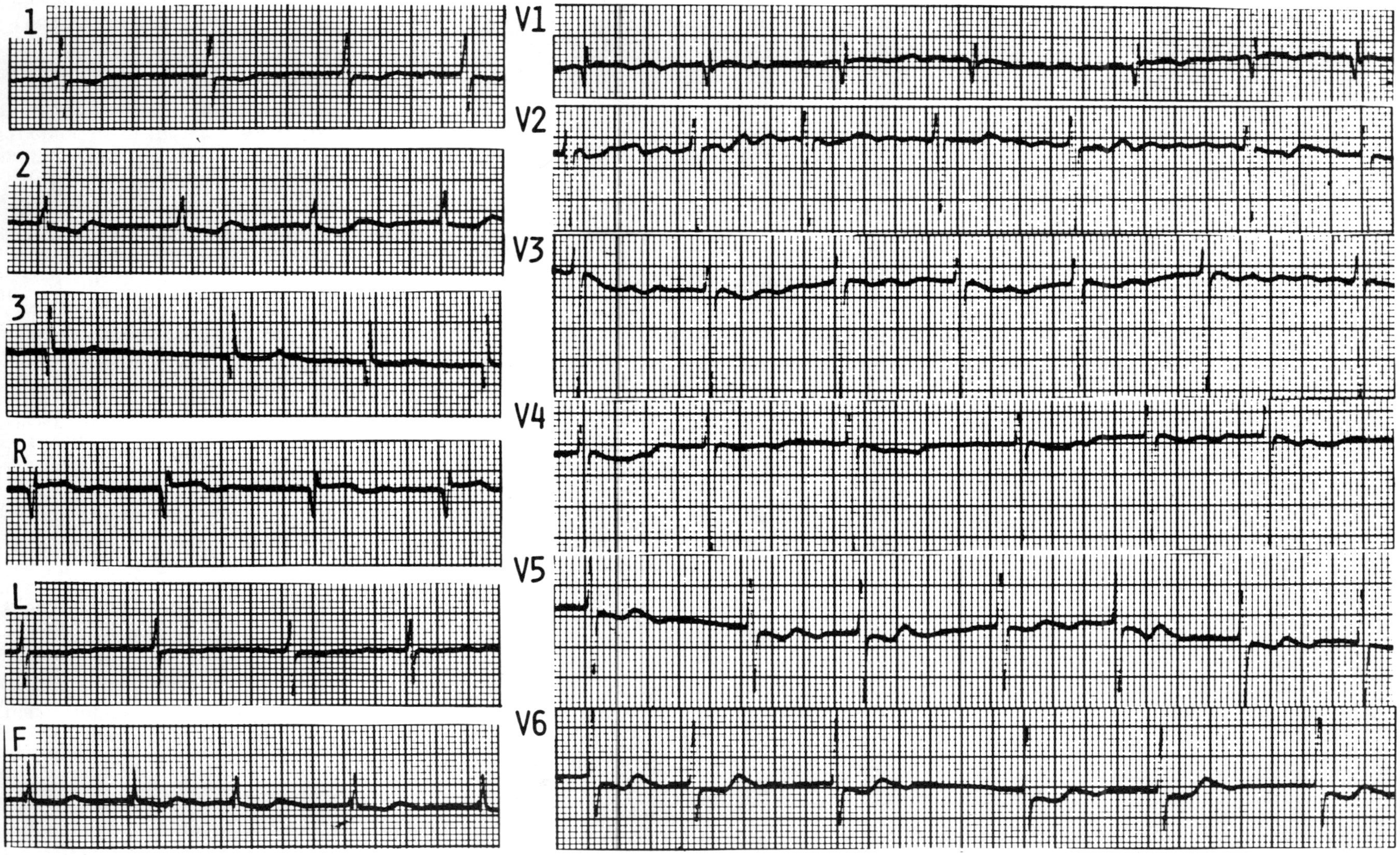


**Figure 11** The 12-lead tracing is of a 70-year-old woman and was taken one day after she was hospitalized for severe, crushing chest pain. Angina pectoris had been present for five years. She was taking digitalis and furosemide orally, and sublingual nitroglycerin.

# NUMBER 11 *See the U-turn?* Jorge I. Martinez-Lopez

## ELUCIDATION

**Diagnosis**—*Inverted U waves*

Atrial fibrillation is present. The ventricular complexes are of normal duration, indicating normal intraventricular conduction of the supraventricular impulses. The QR configuration in $V_1$ and the deep S waves from $V_2$ through $V_6$ are consistent with right ventricular hypertrophy. Most leads display inverted T waves. Inverted U waves occur at fixed intervals from the T waves and are seen best in the precordial leads.

## DISCUSSION

The *U wave* is a small rounded deflection which follows the T wave. If not differentiated from the T wave, it may be confused with a notched T, or lead to erroneous measurement of the QT interval.

Since the description of the *U wave* by Einthoven in 1912, it has received little attention and its genesis has remained both controversial and elusive. Earlier studies attributed the *U wave* either to the development of negative afterpotentials in the ventricular musculature or to delayed repolarization of certain portions of the ventricles. More recently, indirect evidence presented by Watanabe supports the theory that Purkinje repolarization causes the *U wave.*

Normally, the *U wave* has the same polarity as the T wave, but only 5% to 50% of its amplitude, and is largest in leads $V_2$ and $V_3$. It is most prominent with slow heart rates, becoming imperceptible at rates above 90.

While the genesis of the *U wave* is still obscure, its diagnostic value has come into clearer focus. Three basic abnormalities have been described: a) *U wave* alternans; b) alterations in voltage or amplitude; and c) changes in polarity. These may occur as an isolated finding or in association with other electrocardiographic abnormalities.

*U wave* alternans—with or without pulsus alternans—induced by ventricular extrasystoles has been observed and proposed as an "electrocardiographic sign of left ventricular failure."

Voltage of the *U wave* is increased by conditions leading to increased ventricular filling and stroke volume, including bradyarrhythmia, hypopotassemia, in the first beat after any pause in the cardiac cycle, and during coronary angiography. Contrariwise, reduced voltage may result when venous return to the heart and stroke volume are decreased.

Negative (inverted) *U waves* are virtually always associated with heart disease. *Isolated* inversion may appear infrequently as an early manifestation of acute myocardial infarction prior to the demonstration of other ECG abnormalities, as well as in left ventricular hypertrophy or conditions invariably leading to it, angina pectoris, or both. In association with other ECG alterations, negative *U waves* have been observed in right and left ventricular systolic and diastolic overloads, myocardial infarction, papillary muscle disease, and subarachnoid hemorrhage. Although the polarity of the *U wave* is usually the same as that of the T wave, it may not be concordant with the T wave in ventricular extrasystoles and bundle-branch block.

Polarity and voltage of *U waves* should be viewed as dynamic rather than static. This dynamism may reflect improvement or worsening of the clinical situation. For instance, the response of the *U wave* to exercise testing may be of diagnostic value. The normal *U wave* always becomes more positive. The appearance of a negative *U wave* during or after exercise is suggestive of myocardial ischemia, even if no other abnormalities appear. In patients with systemic arterial hypertension, a negative *U wave* can become upright when the blood pressure is reduced by therapy. Inverted *U waves* appear transiently following pulmonary embolism or may become upright after surgical correction of mitral valve disease.

It was mentioned earlier that the *U wave* must be differentiated from the T wave in order to avoid errors in interpretation. This may be difficult to accomplish in situations where the *U wave* appears early or when the QT interval is prolonged, leading to *T-U fusion.* Under such circumstances, this distinction can usually be established by using a nomogram devised by Lepeschkin or simultaneously recording the ECG with a phonocardiogram.

## SELECTED READINGS

Eyer KM: U wave alternans: an electrocardiographic sign of left ventricular failure. *Am Heart J* 87:41–45, 1974.

Lepeschkin E: The U wave of the electrocardiogram. *Mod Concepts Cardiovasc Dis* 38:39–45, 1969.

Watanabe Y: Purkinje repolarization as a possible cause of the U wave in the electrocardiogram. *Circulation* 51:1030–1037, 1975.

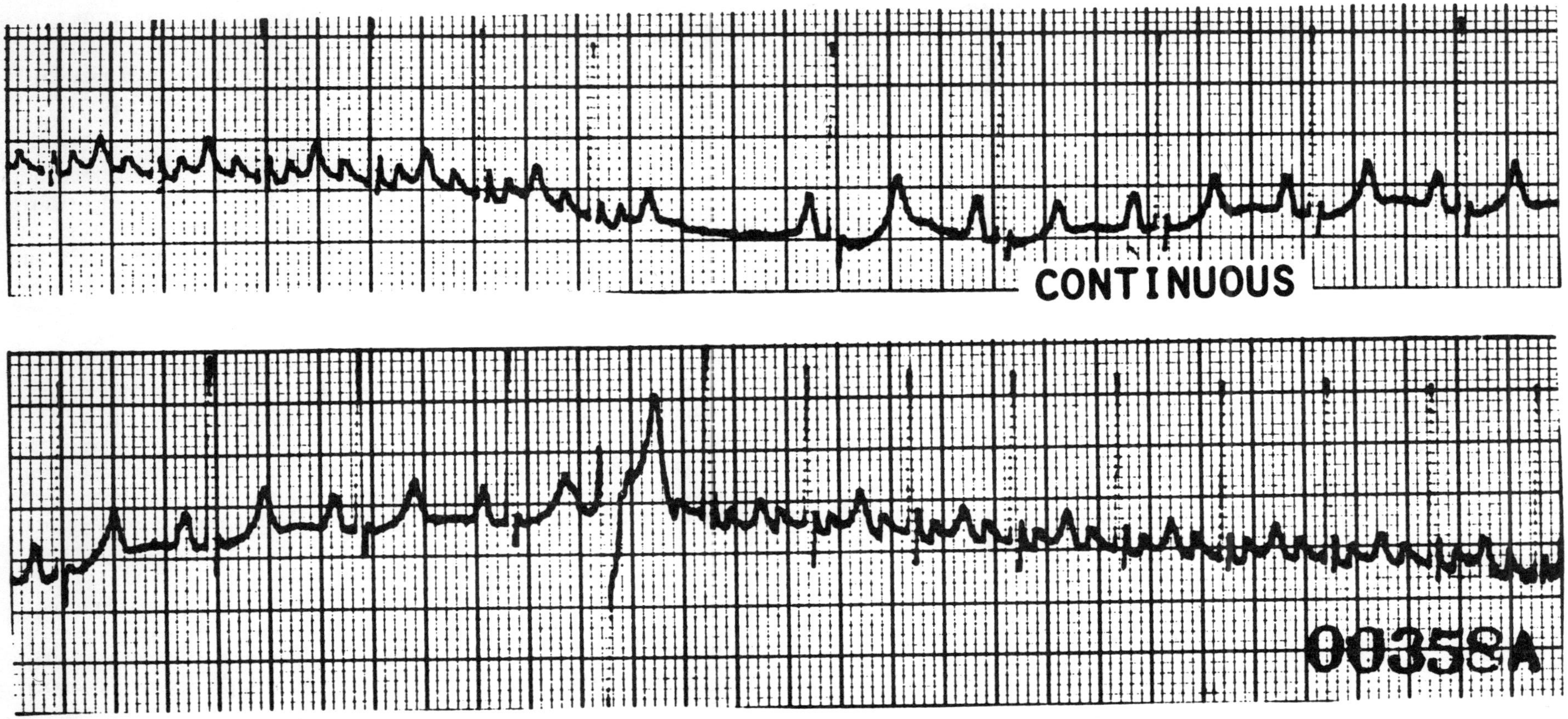


**Figure 12** The tracing is a continuous rhythm strip (lead II) recorded with the Holter monitor. It was taken on a 35-year-old woman with a history of palpitations. She was known to have chronic granulomatous colitis, and was taking sufasalazine, tincture of opium, and prednisone.

# NUMBER 12 *Heart Throbs—Fact or Artifact?* Jorge I. Martinez-Lopez

## ELUCIDATION

**Diagnosis**—*Pseudoarrhythmia due to intermittent recorder motor failure*

The rhythm strip shows several features. The first portion of the top strip shows rapidly occurring, narrow QRS complexes. Sandwiched between flanking QRS complexes are at least four positive waves, which could be erroneously interpreted as "supraventricular tachyarrhythmia with A-V block." This fast sequence ends abruptly by what would appear to be a "blocked atrial beat." After the pause, a slower normal sinus rhythm (72/min) is observed. The QRS complexes are wider, ending with a diminutive secondary "r" wave. T waves are prominent.

On the lower strip, a premature ventricular contraction (PVC) occurs after the fourth normal beat. The premature beat is followed by a recurrence of the faster rate observed earlier.

The transient narrowing and widening of the QRS complexes, P waves, and QT segments, as well as the changes in rate, result from difficulties with the tape driving mechanism.

## DISCUSSION

Continuous ambulatory electrocardiographic monitoring, referred to hereafter as *dynamic electrocardiography* (DCG), is now possible. This technique employs a single bipolar chest lead. The lead wires are attached to a portable, self-contained, battery-powered, magnetic tape recorder carried by the patient. Tracings obtained over extended periods of time may then be scrutinized subsequently, utilizing a rapid playback device. For detailed analysis, suspicious portions of the tracing are selected for printout on standard ECG paper at normal speed (25 mm/sec).

DCG has gained wide acceptance because of the variety of clinical situations in which it may provide valuable information. For instance, DCG is of inestimable value in documenting ECG correlates of symptoms suspected to be of cardiac origin, such as dyspnea, palpitations, chest pain or discomfort, faintness, and syncopal episodes. For such correlation to be possible, however, it is extremely important to have the patient keep an accurate and carefully timed diary of his activities—including smoking, eating, and driving—and symptoms experienced throughout the recording period.

Other indications for DCG include: a) detection of transient asymptomatic arrhythmias and conduction disturbances; b) assessment of the natural history, severity, and physiologic correlates of cardiac arrhythmias in various conditions; c) diagnosis of ischemic heart disease; d) evaluation of the efficacy of antiarrhythmic and antianginal therapy; and e) evaluation of function of artificial cardiac pacemakers.

Despite the abundance of electrophysiologic data that DCG can compile for analysis, the technique is not without inherent problems. Therefore, the physician interpreting such tracings must be expert, not only in the recognition of arrhythmias and conduction disturbances, but also have the knowledge and the ability to recognize artifacts and to differentiate these from true abnormalities. Failure to make this distinction is potentially dangerous, as it enhances the possibility of an erroneous diagnosis which may lead to aggressive and unnecessary therapy.

Artifacts can occur at any point in the monitoring sequence, from the time the leads are attached to the chest wall until the final interpretation is rendered. Careful technique in preparing the skin, careful attachment and positioning of chest leads, and checking for broken lead wires can reduce or eliminate some artifacts.

During the recording period, artifacts may be introduced by intermittent changes in tape speed resulting from battery or motor failure, by frequency response disturbance, and by reusing an incompletely erased tape. Artifacts have also been noted during playback, the major culprits being tape reversal and tape adhering to the scanning head.

Two major forms of artifacts have been described: *pseudoarrhythmias* and *nonarrhythmias.* In the first category, artifacts can mimic atrial and ventricular tachycardia, fusion beats, atrial fibrillation, junctional rhythm, A-V block, and sinus arrest.

In contrast to the pseudoarrhythmias, the nonarrhythmic artifacts seldom create therapeutic hazards. The main danger posed by misinterpretation of these artifacts is the tendency to overestimate their clinical significance. The nonarrhythmic artifacts include aberrancy, low voltage, electrical alternans, ST-segment and T-wave changes, and mirror-image printouts.

It behooves every physician analyzing DCG tracings to have a high index of suspicion and to assume that *all* abnormalities detected by this technique are artifactual until proven otherwise. *Caveat medicus!*

## SELECTED READINGS

Bleifer SB, Bleifer DJ, Hansmann DR, et al: Diagnosis of occult arrhythmias by Holter electrocardiography. *Prog Cardiovasc Dis* 16:569–599, 1974.

Krasnow AZ, Bloomfield DK: Artifacts in portable electrocardiographic monitoring. *Am Heart J* 91:349–357, 1976.

Romero CA Jr: Holter monitoring in the diagnosis and management of cardiac rhythm disturbances. *Med Clin North Am* 60:299–313, 1976.

## **NUMBER 13** *To Pace or Not to Pace* Jorge I. Martinez-Lopez

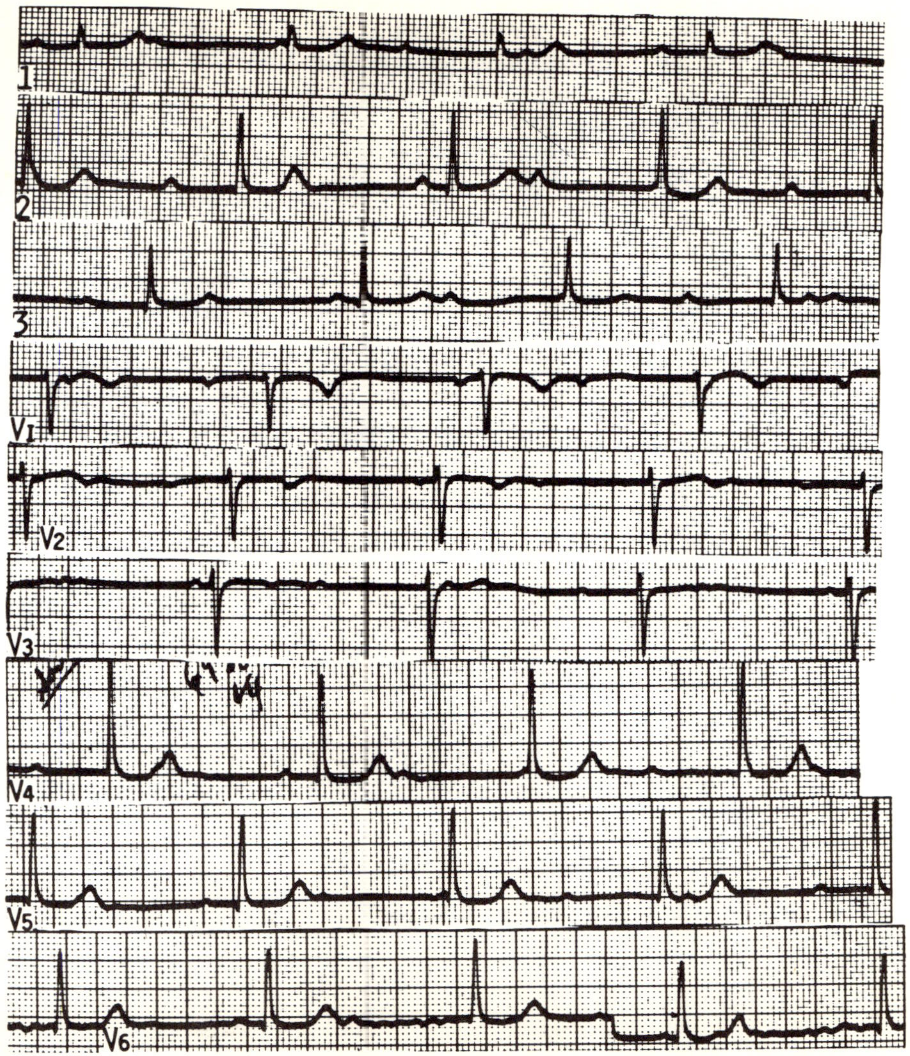


**Figure 13** The tracing was taken on a 24-year-old woman hospitalized at full term with her first pregnancy. She had no symptoms referable to the cardiovascular system. She delivered a live infant subsequently without any difficulty.

# NUMBER 13 *To Pace or Not to Pace* Jorge I. Martinez-Lopez

## ELUCIDATION

**Diagnosis**—*Congenital complete heart block (CCHB)*

The tracing shows complete atrioventricular (AV) dissociation due to complete AV block. The atrial rate is regular at 75/min and the ventricular rate is 45/min. Ventricular complexes occur with regularity and are unrelated to atrial activity. The QRS complexes are narrow, indicating that block is proximal to the bundle of His and that a junctional pacemaker is driving the ventricles. Artifacts are noted in leads $V_1$ and $V_6$.

## DISCUSSION

The etiology of CCHB has not been completely clarified. However, evidence accumulated indicates that in many cases structural abnormalities in the conduction tissue are responsible. Lesions such as absence of the AV node (AVN) or a portion of the bundle of His (BH), destruction by scarring of an area surrounding AVN or BH (from in utero infection?), and isolated tumor involving BH have been described. In some cases CCHB may be a familial disorder; inheritance may be sex-linked. Females are more frequently affected with the disorder than males.

The conduction disturbance may be detected before, at, or soon after birth. Yater's criteria for establishing the diagnosis of CCHB include: 1) graphic evidence of AV block first noted early in life; 2) evidence of existence of slow pulse present at an early age; 3) absence of any preexisting conditions which might cause block after birth, such as rheumatic fever, syphilis, myocarditis, digitalis toxicity, fibroelastosis, etc; and 4) history of syncopal attacks at an early age. All this is fairly good evidence for the presence of block prior to the attack.

The disorder is most frequently seen as an isolated entity but it may be associated with congenital cardiac malformations, including corrected transposition of the great vessels, left-to-right shunts, semilunar valve stenosis, etc.

In the vast majority of cases the subsidiary pacemaker is at the N-H or BH level, and ventricular depolarization follows a normal sequence. The resting ventricular rate remains rather constant during childhood and adulthood at 40–80/minute. It may fall below 40 in the presence of a superimposed cardiac disorder. Exercise and other severe physical stresses generally result in significant increase of ventricular rate, but it is unusual for the rate to exceed 100–130/minute even with severe exercise.

In isolated CCHB, hemodynamic changes represent the effects on the circulation of the conduction disturbance alone, without the underlying myocardial dysfunction generally encountered in acquired heart block or with associated congenital cardiac disease. The cardiac output is usually maintained at normal limits, despite the low heart rate, by an increased stroke volume. Such patients display normal or near normal working capacity and may tolerate high levels of physical exertion without difficulty. Although the reported incidence of Stokes-Adams syndrome varies from 0% to 8%, serious cardiac symptomatology is uncommon. Conversely, manifestations present in patients with associated congenital cardiac or major vascular anomalies are dependent primarily upon the coexisting cardiovascular abnormality.

Since the adverse circulatory hemodynamic effects seen with superimposed heart disease (congenital or acquired) are not seen in isolated CCHB, ventricular pacing (temporary or permanent) is *not* indicated unless major cardiac symptoms or evidence of electrical instability is present.

# NUMBER 14 *Ventricular Ectopy—Benign or Malignant?* Jorge I. Martinez-Lopez

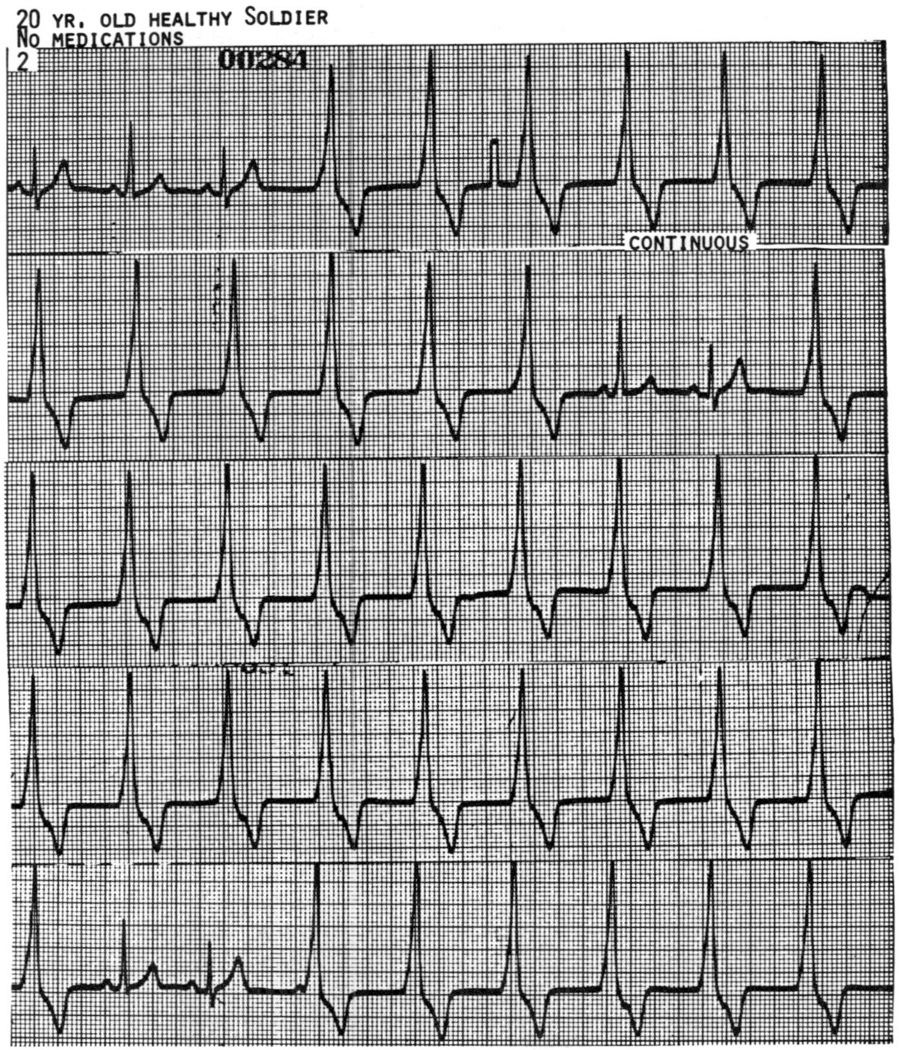


**Figure 14** The rhythm strip (lead II) is of a 20-year-old soldier with vague complaints and no known previous history of heart disease. The physical examination was entirely normal except for intermittent abnormal splitting of the second heart sound. He was on no medications.

# NUMBER 14 *Ventricular Ectopy—Benign or Malignant?* Jorge I. Martinez-Lopez

## ELUCIDATION

**Diagnosis**—*Accelerated idioventricular rhythm (AIVR)*

At the beginning of the tracing the first three beats show a normal sinus rhythm (NSR). The second QRS complex, however, is slightly different from the flanking, normal QRS complexes, and represents a fusion beat. The fourth through fifteenth beats are bizarre in appearance, longer in duration, are not preceded by P waves, and are followed by secondary ST-T changes. These complexes represent the accelerated ventricular escape rhythm which becomes manifest when the sinus rhythm slows down. A fusion beat is again seen in the transition period from AIVR or NSR. Subsequently, several episodes of AIVR recur. In the bottom strip, the fourth beat is preceded by a P wave, which is obviously not conducted.

## DISCUSSION

Accelerated idioventricular rhythm is *not* indicative of heart disease. It may be observed in otherwise healthy subjects or in association with heart disease. The reported incidence in acute myocardial infarction varies from 16% to 36%. Also, AIVR may be an expression of toxicity in patients taking digitalis.

The arrhythmia represents a sustained, *passive* ventricular rhythm which, although ectopic in origin, is *benign* in nature. The QRS complexes are abnormal in shape and duration, with secondary ST-T changes. The ventricular rate varies from 50/minute to 100/minute and is regular. Most commonly, the ectopic center is unifocal, but it may be multifocal. Transient isorhythmic AV dissociation occurs when AIVR becomes manifest. Fusion beats are common and represent transitional ventricular complexes.

Ordinarily, the fastest pacemaker is in control of the heart. Consequently, slower subsidiary pacemakers are suppressed and kept from firing spontaneously. Ventricular arrhythmias may become manifest when the dominant pacemaker fails to depolarize the ventricles or when the ectopic focus becomes the fastest pacemaker. Hence, circumstances which may promote the appearance of AIVR include: a) disturbances of impulse conduction, such as SA and AV block; b) disturbances of impulse formation, such as marked sinus bradycardia or sinus arrest; c) when the inherent rate of the ventricular focus exceeds that of the normally firing SA node; and d) combinations of the above.

The major clinical distinction is between AIVR and true ventricular tachycardia and junctional rhythm with aberrant conduction. Less frequently, AIVR may be confused with premature ventricular beats and ventricular parasystole. Although the surface electrocardiogram is extremely useful in differentiating these arrhythmias, bundle of His electrograms may be necessary to determine whether AIVR or junctional rhythm with aberrant conduction is present.

The treatment of AIVR in the absence of heart disease is "masterly inactivity", for the condition is hemodynamically insignificant and does not pose the threat of more serious arrhythmias. Rarely is active treatment indicated, even when heart disease coexists. However, AIVR may need to be abolished when there are adverse hemodynamic effects resulting from loss of atrial contribution or from a fast ventricular rate. Otherwise, treatment is directed at the underlying cardiac disorder. Though transient AV dissociation does occur during AIVR, it must not be confused with complete heart block. Therefore, cardiac pacing is not indicated.

## SELECTED READINGS


Lichstein E, et al: Incidence and description of accelerated ventricular rhythm complicating acute myocardial infarction. *Am J Med* 58:192–198, 1975.

Massumi RA, Ali N: Accelerated isorhythmic ventricular rhythms. *Am J Cardiol* 26:170–185, 1970.

Rothfeld EL, Zucher IR: Multiform accelerated idioventricular rhythm. *Angiology* 25:457–461, 1974.

Schamroth L: Idioventricular tachycardia. *J Electrocardiol* 1:205–212, 1968.

## NUMBER 15 *Dissolving the Association* Jorge I. Martinez-Lopez

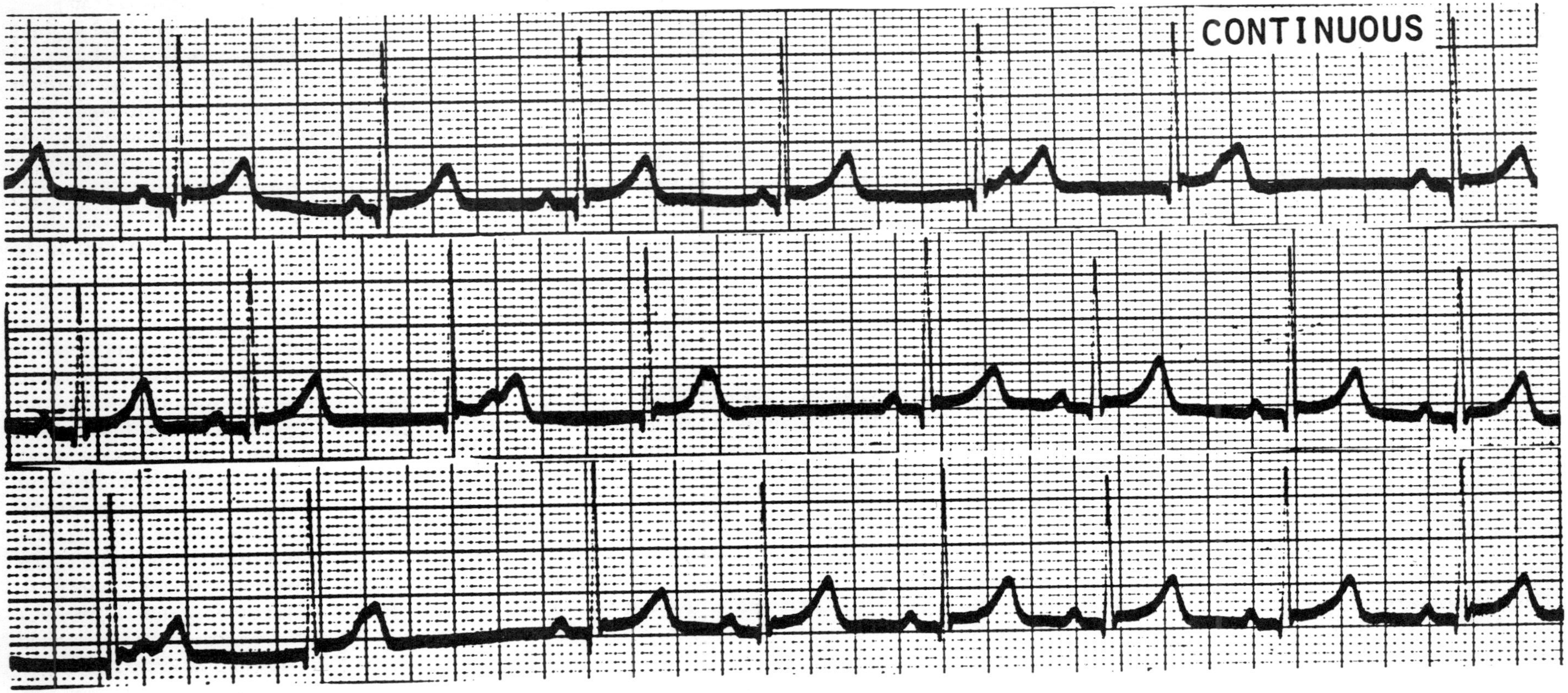


**Figure 15** This rhythm strip (lead II) is of a 14-year-old girl who was found to have a basal systolic ejection murmur. She was on no medications.

# NUMBER 15 *Dissolving the Association* Jorge I. Martinez-Lopez

## ELUCIDATION

**Diagnosis**—*AV dissociation*

Normal sinus rhythm and normal intraventricular conduction are noted. In the top strip, the prominent feature is the gradual "moving in" of the P wave toward the QRS complexes, and then reappearing in front of the QRS. This sequence recurs throughout the remainder of the tracing and is related to respiration.

Hence, for a few cardiac cycles there is transient AV dissociation when the P-P interval widens (ie, when the sinoatrial rate slows down). Under such conditions, the sinus node remains in control of the atria, but the junctional area is quick to intervene, providing the spark necessary to initiate ventricular depolarization. Accordingly, the R-R intervals of the dissociated beats are also wider (ie, the ventricular rate is slower, but faster than the atrial rate).

## DISCUSSION

The term "AV dissociation" is a common source of confusion among inexperienced electrocardiographic interpreters, being poorly understood by many, improperly used by others, and misinterpreted by still others.

It is essential to have a precise interpretation because there are many forms of AV dissociation and they are not managed in identical manner. It follows that treatment—and whether it is necessary or not—is dictated by the type of AV dissociation, among other factors.

*AV dissociation* (AVD) means that the atria and the ventricles have dissolved their temporal association, ie, that they beat independently of each other. In the presence of AVD, when there is a conducted beat—even once—dissociation is *incomplete;* when none are conducted, it is *complete.* Hence, the atria and ventricles are under control of separate pacemakers for one or more cardiac cycles, and P waves and QRS complexes do not have a constant temporal relationship on the ECG during such periods.

It is important for the interpreter to understand that AVD is "never a primary disturbance of rhythm....but rather the consequence of some other basic disorder." This simply means that the term is no more specific than such terms as "cyanosis," "jaundice," "anemia," or "heart failure." Therefore, it is imperative that, once AVD has been established as the arrhythmia, its exact cause be determined.

As already stated, AVD is the end result of other primary cardiac rhythm disorders. Some of these are physiologic in nature while others are induced by pharmacologic agents or by pathologic changes in the heart. The *major causes* are: a) slowing of the primary pacemaker, the SA node; b) acceleration of secondary pacemakers in the junctional area or ventricles; c) AV conduction disturbances; d) electrical pacing of the ventricle; and e) combinations of the above.

The case presented here represents an example of incomplete AVD resulting from intermittent slowing of the SA node induced by respiration (sinus arrhythmia), requiring no therapy. At the time of AVD, the atria remained under control of the SA node, while the ventricles were driven by stimuli originating in the junctional area. This junctional rhythm is in this instance *passive,* arising *by default* as a "rescue" mechanism. This form of AVD and that seen in sinus bradycardia may occur in perfectly healthy young adults without any evidence of heart disease. On the other hand, slowing of the SA node resulting in AVD may be secondary to the administration of pharmacologic agents with negative chronotropic effects (eg, rauwolfia, propranolol, etc), and to the presence of underlying heart disease. Sinoatrial arrest, sinoatrial block, and the "sick-sinus syndrome" are virtually always a result of serious heart disease, and management is determined by the cause of the arrhythmia, by the presence of symptoms, and by the type of heart disease present.

In the second type of AVD, the firing rate of the SA node is normal, but the junctional area or the ventricle *actively* initiates impulses at a rate faster than the SA node. Such bursts may be either paroxysmal or nonparoxysmal. In either case, the rhythm established *usurps* the role of the SA node and controls the ventricles. Examples are junctional and ventricular tachycardia. In the latter, supraventricular impulses may be occasionally "captured" by the junctional area and conducted antegrade to the ventricles, resulting in normalization of the QRS complex. This beat, when recorded, is referred to as a *Dressler's beat* and is pathognomonic of ventricular tachycardia.

Advanced or complete AV block represents the third type of AVD. In the former, AVD is incomplete; in the latter, complete. Either one may be transient or permanent. Complete AV block may be congenital or acquired.

Use of ventricular pacing—whether epicardial or endocardial—also results in AVD. In this circumstance, the atria may be under SA node dominance or under control of supraventricular ectopic centers such as in atrial tachycardia, flutter, or fibrillation; the ventricular musculature, by the electrical stimulus emanating from the artificial pacemaker. Whether AVD is complete or incomplete is determined by the type of pacemaker used (demand *vs* fixed-type), by the nature of the supraventricular mechanism, and by the integrity (conductance) of the junctional area.

## SELECTED READINGS

Chung EK: Atrioventricular dissociation revisited. *Cardiol Digest* June 1973, pp 29–37.

Marriott HJL, Menendez MM: AV dissociation revisited. *Prog Cardiovasc Dis* 8:522–538, 1966.

Pick A: AV dissociation: a proposal for a comprehensive classification and consistent terminology. *Am Heart J* 66:147–150, 1963.

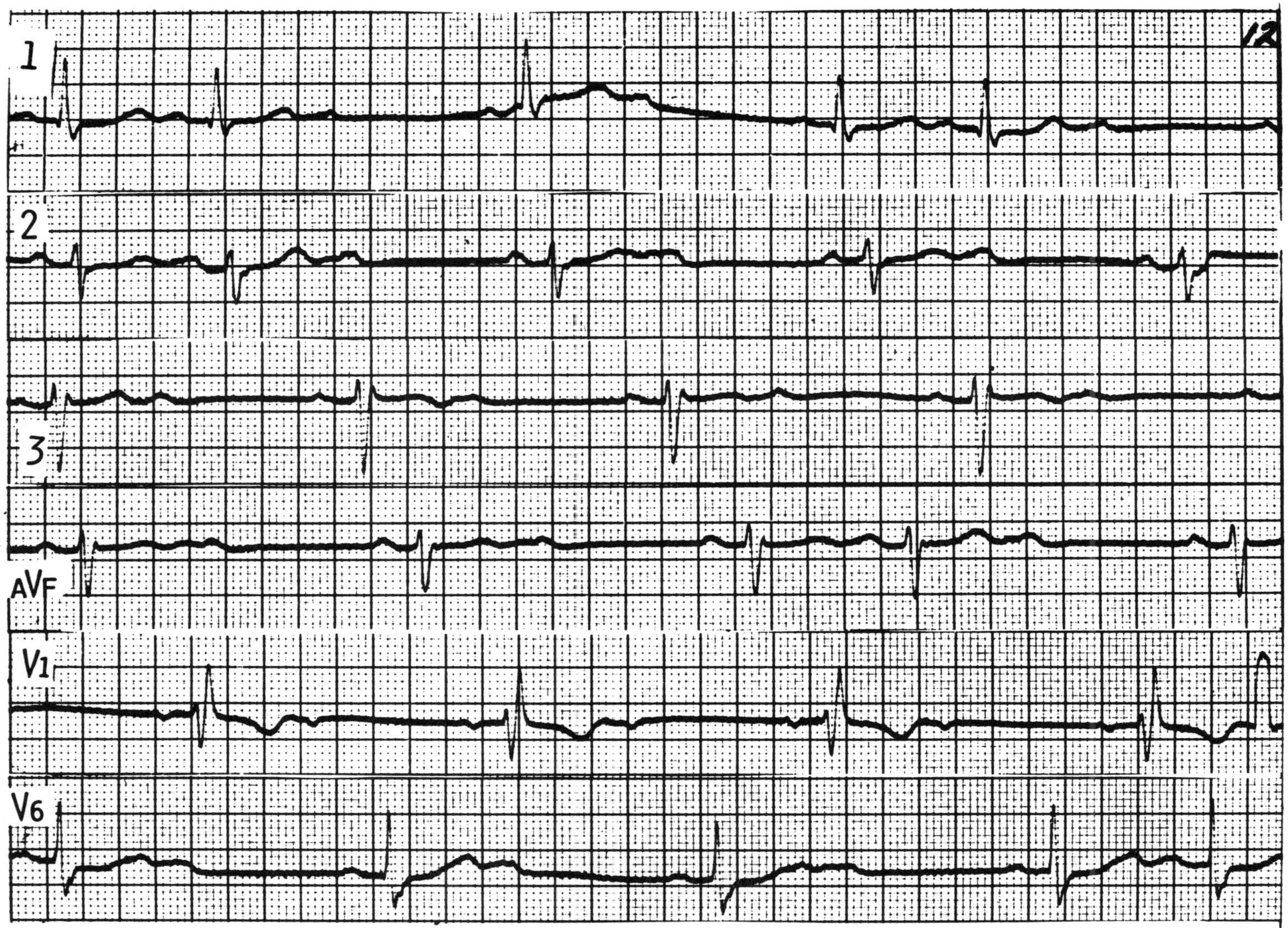


**Figure 16** The tracing is of a 74-year-old woman seen in consultation because of repeated episodes of dizziness and near-syncope, originally attributed to "middle ear disease." The leads were not taken simultaneously.

# NUMBER 16 *The Pause That Distresses* Jorge I. Martinez-Lopez

## ELUCIDATION

**Diagnosis**—*Second-degree AV block (Mobitz type II)*

Normal sinus rhythm is present. The P-R interval of the conducted beats is constant and at upper normal limits. The QRS complexes are abnormal in duration (0.12 sec) and display a right bundle branch block pattern. Abnormal deviation of the electrical axis to the left is observed in the frontal leads.

The prominent feature is the presence of nonconducted sinus impulses in 3:2 and 2:1 AV ratios. The nonconducted impulses occur unexpectedly and are followed by lengthy pauses, causing the effective ventricular rate to drop drastically.

The electrocardiographic diagnosis is: second-degree AV block (Mobitz type II), with left anterior fascicular block, and complete right bundle branch block.

## DISCUSSION

Traditional concepts of intraventricular conduction were revolutionized when Rosenbaum and associates introduced the trifascicularity of the intraventricular conduction system. Basically, their scheme proposed that the electrical excitation process of the heart reached the ventricles over a three-pronged system: the right bundle branch, and the anterior and posterior fascicles of the left bundle branch.

More recent anatomic studies indicate that the intraventricular conduction network does not ramify in such a simplistic manner, that not all of the fascicles are so clearly defined, and that there are vast amounts of interfascicular connections. Nevertheless, from the electrophysiologic viewpoint, there is merit to the concepts proposed by Rosenbaum et al. Variability in the site of major lesions within the trifascicular conduction system and the progressive nature of the conduction disturbances lead to a variety of ECG patterns.

Second-degree AV block is a conduction disturbance in which not every sinus impulse is propagated into the ventricles. It is subclassified into type I (Wenckebach periodicity), type II, and advanced block. The conduction disorder is expressed as a conduction ratio of the number of supraventricular impulses to the number of ventricular repsonses. The discussion which follows is limited to type II.

In type II AV block, the intermittent failure of sinus impulses to enter and depolarize the ventricles leads to pauses, the lengths of which are determined by when the next conducted sinus impulse is formed or by whether or not escape impulses or other ectopic rhythms emerge during the pause. Sequences of nonconducted sinus impulses can occur with a *fixed* AV ratio (2:1 or other) or with a *varying* AV ratio (2:1, 3:2, etc). In contrast to type I AV block, the P-R interval remains constant in those sinus impulses which are conducted. Because type II block derives from lesions below the bundle of His, involving at least two of the three fascicles, the QRS complexes are abnormal both in duration and configuration. Ventricular complexes most commonly display a right bundle branch block pattern. Infrequently, alternating right and left bundle branch block are recorded in the same tracing. If the location of the block is above the bundle of His, the QRS complexes are normal in duration; this pattern is seldom observed. Finally, deviations in the electrical axis in the frontal plane reflect the involvement of the left-sided fascicles. In general, abnormal left axis deviation indicates left anterior fascicular block, while right axis deviation implies block in the territory of the left posterior fascicle.

Type II AV block is viewed as a prelude to complete heart block. The electrocardiographic abnormalities develop insidiously, and may progress either gradually or remain relatively stable. For these reasons, the surface ECG cannot be used to predict when complete heart block will occur or to provide clues as to the cause of type II block.

The ECG abnormalities seen in type II block virtually always precede the onset of symptoms. Therefore, when the patient is first seen, symptoms may or may not be present. Once type II block has been uncovered, it is important to obtain a very thorough history in an attempt to unearth symptoms which, however subtle, may be cardiac-related. Equally important is to carry out long-term ambulatory monitoring on magnetic tape (Holter). This is done also to assess the "stability" or "instability" of the observed block.

Symptoms, when present, are related to

the basic heart rate, to the pause occasioned by the nonconducted sinus impulse, and to whether or not other ectopic rhythms ensue during the pause. In many cases, the vague symptomatology is ascribed to noncardiac disorders. Dizziness, greying-out episodes, syncope, and Stokes-Adams-Morgagni episodes form part of the spectrum of the presenting transient neurologic manifestations, alone or in combination.

With the development of effective treatment, ie, artificial cardiac pacemaker, the diagnosis of second-degree, type II AV block has assumed increased importance. In general, controversy persists regarding the management of *asymptomatic* patients. Bundle of His recordings are advocated by some authorities to resolve the issue. They recommend permanent pacemaker implantation in those patients in whom the H-V interval is prolonged. Recent studies and an editorial contradict such recommendations.

There is general agreement that in the presence of symptoms caused by the block, permanent implantation of a cardiac pacemaker is indicated. And, in the absence of dysfunction of the SA node, pacemakers sensing sinus impulses and firing in the ventricle in response to them are preferable because they behave more physiologically: responding to changes in sinus rates, and improving cardiac output and stroke volume by coupling ventricular responses with the booster action of the atria.

The patient presented here was clearly symptomatic, but her symptoms initially were not considered to be cardiogenic. Discovery of the type II block led to hospitalization, insertion of a temporary pacemaker and, later, implantation of a permanent pacemaker. Electrophysiologic studies* clearly demonstrated blockage of the nonconducted sinus impulses below the bundle of His, as well as absent retrograde VA conduction. Because evidence for sinus dysfunction was lacking, a programmable, P-wave synchronized pacer was implanted. Symptoms disappeared.

## SELECTED READINGS

Denes P, Dhingra RC, et al: H-V interval in patients with bifascicular block (right bundle branch block and left anterior hemiblock). *Am J Cardiol* 35:23–29, 1975.

Kastor JA: Hemiblock and stopped hearts. *N Engl J Med* 299:249–251, 1978.

McAnulty JH, Rahimtoola SH, et al: A prospective study of sudden death in "high risk" bundle branch block. *N Engl J Med* 299:209–215, 1978.

Rosenbaum MD, Elizari MV, Lazzari JO: The Hemiblocks. Tampa Tracings, Oldsmar, Fla, 1970.

---

*By Dr. P.J. Bower

## NUMBER 17 *Going My Way* Jorge I. Martinez-Lopez

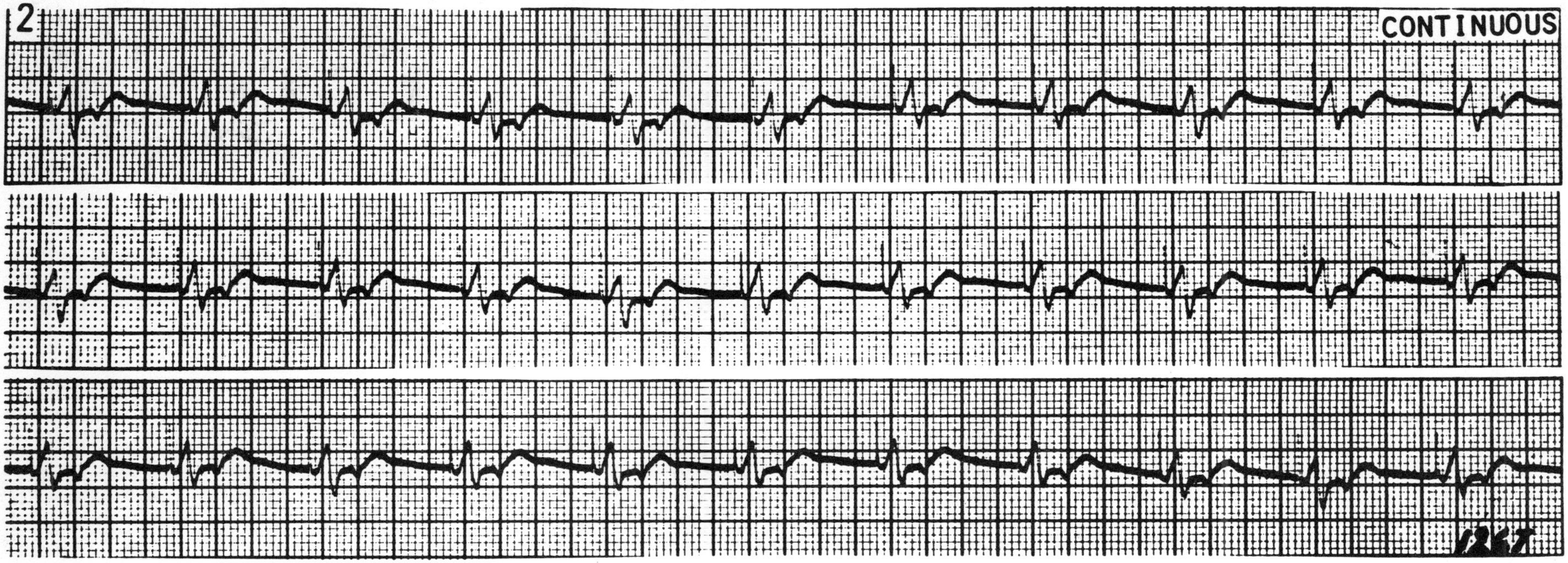


**Figure 17** The rhythm strip is of a 64-year-old woman, admitted to the hospital with diagnoses of diabetes mellitus, pulmonary emphysema, and hypertensive cardiovascular disease complicated by complete AV block. The tracing was taken several days postoperatively. She was taking methyldopa, hydrochlorothiazide, digoxin, tolbutamide, and a potassium supplement.

# NUMBER 17 *Going My Way* Jorge I. Martinez-Lopez

## ELUCIDATION

**Diagnosis**—*Electrical pacing of the ventricle and retrograde VA conduction*

The tracing shows a pacemaker spike immediately preceding every QRS complex (1:1 pacemaker-to-ventricular response). Ventricular complexes are abnormal in duration (0.14 sec), indicating that the chamber paced is the ventricle.

The prominent feature is the presence of *inverted* P′ waves following every paced ventricular complex; the R-P′ interval is approximately 0.22 sec. This sequence establishes the presence of retrograde VA conduction of the paced ventricular impulse into the atria.

## DISCUSSION

The primary function of the conduction system of the heart, from SA node to the Purkinje fibers, is to carry the electrical impulse in an orderly fashion from its proximal source of origin distally to the ventricular musculature; this is termed *anterograde conduction.* Its capacity for *retrograde* conduction to the atria of impulses originating in the AV node, bundle of His, and ventricular automatic cells has also been recognized since the early days of electrocardiography. Hence, electrical impulses in the heart can travel bidirectionally.

Pathologic lesions responsible for complete AV heart block have been found above, at, and/or below the bundle of His; in the majority of cases they are infra-Hisian. It is usually assumed that complete AV block precludes not only anterograde conduction but retrograde (VA) conduction as well. In other words, the observed block is bidirectional.

Retrograde conduction may be partially or totally intact in the presence of complete AV block; ie, there is only *unidirectional* block. This phenomenon has been well documented as a relatively frequent occurrence, having been reported following spontaneous ventricular premature and ventricular automatic beats, and during electrical pacing of the ventricle. It may be either: a) *manifest,* as observed on the surface ECG, or b) *concealed,* and unmasked by intracardiac electrophysiologic studies. Although a variety of mechanisms have been hypothesized, the phenomenon of unidirectional, complete AV block remains unexplained.

The patient presented here showed complete AV block with the spontaneous subsidiary pacemaker located in the ventricle, firing regularly at 20 times per minute. Insertion of a temporary pacemaker was followed by implantation of a permanent artificial pacemaker. Shortly after its implantation, it was observed that every paced ventricular complex was followed by an abnormal P′ wave *(atrial captured beat)* and that the R-P′ interval was short. From this it was deduced that the paced ventricular impulse traveled retrograde into the atria.

The P′ wave in retrograde conduction may precede the QRS complex, be buried in it, or follow it, depending on the location of the ectopic pacemaker and factors influencing conduction. In the presence of atrial captured beats during ventricular pacing, the P′ wave virtually always follows the QRS complex, and the R-P′ interval is of "normal" duration or prolonged. The relatively short R-P′ interval in this patient cannot be explained.

Other variants of retrograde conduction have been reported with less frequency. Progressive lengthening of the R-P′ interval can occur, resulting in retrograde Wenckebach periodicity. Reciprocation may occur in complete AV block *if* there is longitudinal dissociation in the junctional tissues. Atrial captured beats may occur only in alternate paced beats because of impaired conduction ("rate-dependent").

Recognition of retrograde conduction during ventricular pacing is important because it may be erroneously attributed to pacemaker malfunction, leading to unnecessary explanation. Clinically, its recognition is also important because in some patients hemodynamic deterioration and severe disability may result. In such cases, the constant superimposition of atrial and ventricular systole leads to inadequate left ventricular filling, pulmonary congestion, and depressed cardiac output.

## SELECTED READINGS

Cohen SI, et al: Concealed retrograde conduction in complete atrioventricular block. *Circulation* 50:496, 1974.

Gupta PK, Haft JI: Retrograde ventriculoatrial

**NUMBER 17** *Going My Way* Jorge I. Martinez-Lopez

conduction in complete heart block: studies with His bundle electrography. *Am J Cardiol* 30:408, 1972.

Johnson AD, et al: Hemodynamic compromise associated with ventriculoatrial conduction following transvenous pacemaker placement. *Am J Med* 65:75, 1978.

Khalilullah M, et al: Unidirectional complete heart block. *Am Heart J* 97:608, 1979.

# NUMBER 18 *Take-off or Put-on?* Jorge I. Martinez-Lopez

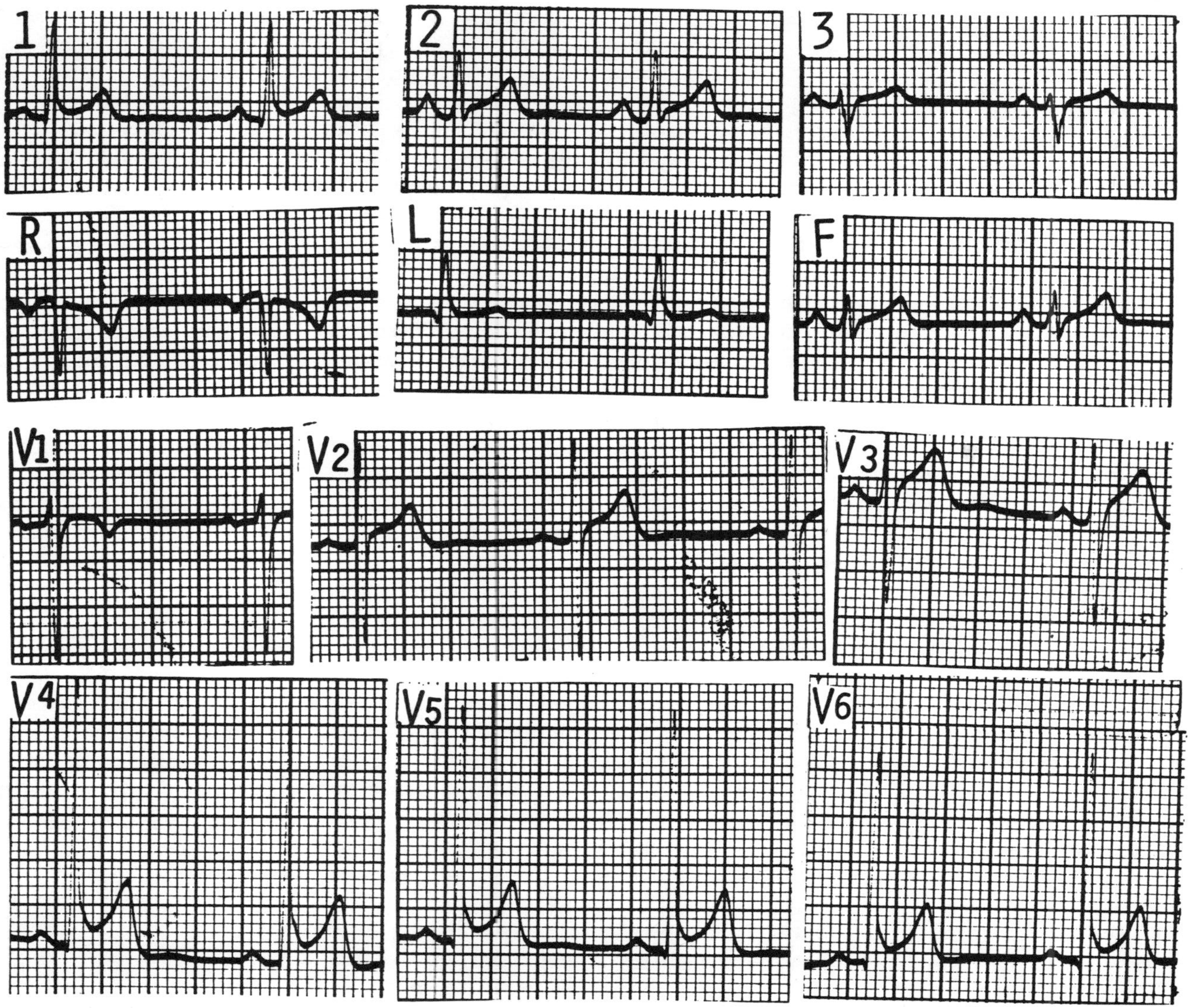


**Figure 18** This preoperative 12-lead tracing is of a 27-year-old man hospitalized following a gunshot wound to the face. He was on no medications.

# NUMBER 18 *Take-off or Put-on?* Jorge I. Martinez-Lopez

## ELUCIDATION

**Diagnosis**—*Early repolarization syndrome*

Normal sinus rhythm is present. The prominent feature is the elevated ST segments in limb leads I and II and in the precordial leads from $V_3$ through $V_6$. In addition, tall R waves and peaked T waves are present from $V_4$ through $V_6$. The tracing is a *normal variant.*

## DISCUSSION

Considerable importance is ascribed to deviations of the ST segment in the electrocardiogram. *Elevation* is most frequently due to an epicardial current of injury resulting from ischemic heart disease (eg, Prinzmetal's angina) or from inflammatory or neoplastic disorders involving the pericardium and/or the myocardium. Less frequent causes include hyperkalemia, cerebrovascular accidents, and hypothermia.

For over four decades, it has been recognized that ST-segment elevation may also be found in the electrocardiograms of approximately 2% of the normal, adult population. The frequency with which it is observed may be affected, to some extent, by the physical characteristics of the recording machine. This *benign* form of ST-segment elevation, a physiologic variant, is commonly referred to as the "early repolarization syndrome"; the deviation of the ST segment is termed "high take-off." Male predominance has been noted. Racial predilection has not been clearly established, although some believe the syndrome to be more common in young, adult blacks.

Recognition of the syndrome, which depends largely on awareness of its existence and on experience, is important because the observed patterns simulate acute myocardial injury. Conversely, on occasion, ST-segment changes of epicardial injury may mimic the features of early repolarization. Consequently, a thorough history and physical examination, *serial electrocardiograms,* and other ancillary laboratory data may be necessary to assess the significance of the tracings.

"High take-off" of the ST segment in the "early repolarization syndrome" most often persists for many decades, though there is a tendency to decrease with age. Less often, the deviation of the ST segment is observed intermittently, particularly in the left precordial leads. Maximal elevation of the ST segment rarely exceeds 4 mm, with most instances occurring between 0.5 mm and 2.0 mm. In general, the elevated ST segment is most frequent in the anterolateral precordial leads alone, or in combination with one or more limb leads. Rarely, it is noted in the right precordial leads alone. Isolated elevation of ST segments in the limb leads (with normal precordial leads) is also uncommon. Reciprocal ST-segment depression may or may not occur in $aV_R$; elevation in this lead has not been reported.

There are other associated electrocardiographic changes. Tall, peaked, slightly asymmetrical T waves are frequently recorded in leads displaying "high take-off" of the ST segments. Less often, so-called "juvenile" T-wave patterns and "isolated T-wave negativity syndrome" are found. High voltage R waves in lateral precordial leads, mimicking left ventricular hypertrophy, occur frequently. Prominent U waves are seldom seen.

Subjects exhibiting this electrocardiographic syndrome are asymptomatic, show no evidence of detectable heart disease, and have an excellent prognosis. Therapy and limitation of activities are, therefore, not necessary.

A final comment. In analyzing tracings, the interpreter must also take into consideration spurious elevation of the ST segment. For instance, artifactual elevation can occur with an overdamped stylus. Apparent, rather than real, elevation of the ST segment may be the result of a prominent wave of atrial repolarization ($T_a$ wave) which extends beyond the QRS complex or due to downward displacement of the P-R segment secondary to either atrial infarction or atrial pacing.

## SELECTED READINGS


Kambara H, Phillips J: Long-term evaluation of early repolarization syndrome (normal variant RS-T segment elevation). *Am J Cardiol* 38:157–161, 1976.

Parisi AF, Beckmann CH, Lancaster MC: The spectrum of ST segment elevation in the electrocardiograms of healthy adult men. *J Electrocardiol* 4:137–144, 1971.

Rothfeld EL: The itinerant ST-T segment. *Heart and Lung* 6:857–873, 1977.

# NUMBER 19 *A Sheep in Wolf's Clothing* Jorge I. Martinez-Lopez

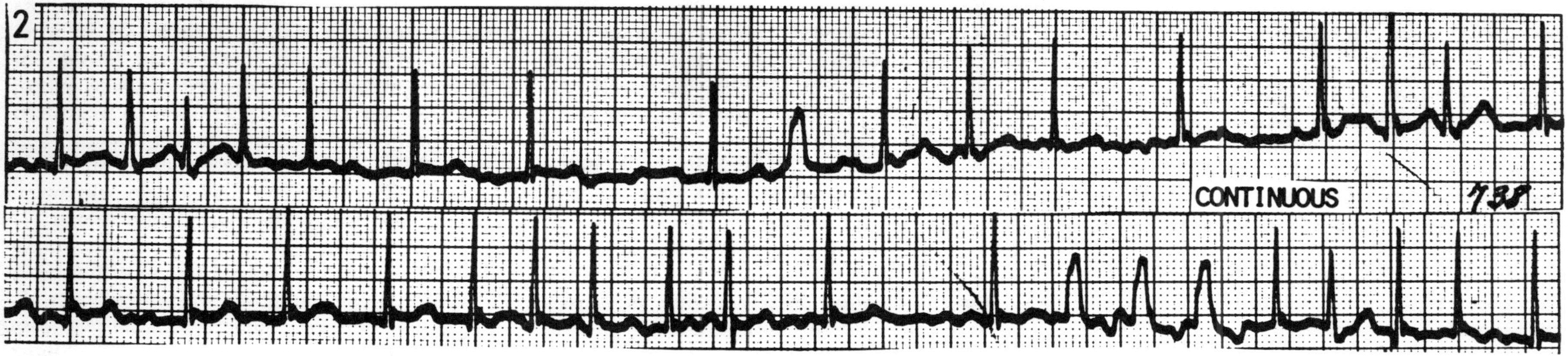


**Figure 19** The rhythm strip was taken in a 47-year-old man admitted with a suspected diagnosis of acute myocardial infarction. On admission, he was taking only chlordiazepoxide hydrochloride.

# NUMBER 19 *A Sheep in Wolf's Clothing* Jorge I. Martinez-Lopez

## ELUCIDATION

**Diagnosis**—*Ashman's phenomenon*

The tracing shows atrial fibrillation with grossly irregular ventricular response. The QRS complexes of the basic rhythm are normal in duration.

Prominent throughout the tracing are ventricular complexes of variable duration and appearance which appear early or very early in relation to the length of the preceding R-R cycle, and which display a nonfixed coupling interval to the preceding R wave. Examine QRS complexes number 3, 9, 15, and 16 on the top strip, and number 9, 12 through 14, 16, and 17 on the bottom strip. These complexes represent aberrant anterograde conduction of the supraventricular impulses and masquerade as either ventricular premature beats or ventricular tachycardia.

## DISCUSSION

Atrial fibrillation (AF) and ventricular premature beats (VPB) are two frequently observed cardiac arrhythmias. Each can occur in the absence of the other, or they can occur concurrently.

In AF, the ventricular rate may be constantly fast or slow, or it may vary. In the absence of complete anterograde block, the ventricular rhythm is totally irregular, and it is impossible to predict when the next conducted ventricular impulse will be recorded on the electrocardiogram. Thus, ventricular complexes will occur early or late in relationship to the preceding R-R cycle.

As long as the ventricular complexes are of normal duration, it can be confidently deduced that they occur in response to stimuli of supraventricular origin. When there is preexisting, established bundle branch block and *all* QRS complexes display the same pattern from beat to beat, the supraventricular origin of the impulse can also be established.

Problems arise when QRS complexes of abnormal duration and configuration appear intermittently in the tracing among the ventricular complexes of the basic rhythm. The questions are: What are they? Are they supraventricular impulses conducted anterograde with aberration or do they represent ventricular ectopy? The answers to these questions have clinical relevance because therapy differs. Misinterpretation of the rhythm diagnosis will lead to an erroneous therapeutic approach. For example, digitalis is often the drug of choice in treating atrial fibrillation *with* or *without* aberrant ventricular conduction. In contrast, lidocaine, quinidine, procainamide, and disopyramide phosphate are frequent drugs of choice in treating VPB or ventricular tachycardia.

How can this dilemma be resolved? The following suggestions are usually helpful in distinguishing between the two. First, take a long rhythm strip, using either $V_1$ or $MCL_1$. A long strip will provide meaningful data, including the morphology of the QRS complexes in question, as well as their relation to the preceding ventricular complex, to the preceding R-R interval, and to the heart rate in general. Second, the diagnosis of VPB is favored by these features: a *fixed* coupling interval; the 0.02-second deflection is different from that of the ventricular complexes of the basic rhythm; the "R-on-T" phenomenon; and, possibly, by "multifocal" beats. Remember that in atrial fibrillation, VPB *are not* followed by a full compensatory pause.

The electrophysiologic basis for aberrantly conducted beats in AF was described by Gouaux and Ashman in 1947: the concept is now designated as the *"Ashman phenomenon."* In a thyrotoxic patient taking quinidine for AF, they recorded aberrant ventricular complexes "when short ventricular cycles follow relatively long cycles, or when very short cycles follow cycles of average length." Variable degrees of aberration were noted, as well as repetitive aberrancy simulating paroxysmal ventricular tachycardia.

The Ashman phenomenon is relatively easy to understand. Aberrancy is apt to occur in AF whenever supraventricular impulses arrive at the ventricular conduction system and find one or more fascicles in a refractory state. Since the right bundle branch is the longest and has a refractory period slightly longer than that of the fascicles of the left bundle branch, the most common pattern recorded is that of a right bundle branch block (rsR′, or rSR′, with a clearly defined S wave). The cycle length, ie, the R-R interval, also plays an important role. In general, when the

R-R interval is prolonged, so is the refractory period of the bundle branches. Therefore, aberrant conduction is favored when a supraventricular impulse arrives *early* at the ventricular conduction system following a long preceding R-R interval, or when it arrives *very early* following an R-R interval of average length.

In exceptional cases, the distinction between aberrancy and ventricular ectopy can be established by the bundle of His electrogram. Simply stated, aberrantly conducted impulses are preceded by a His spike, whereas ventricular ectopy is not.

The "malignant" appearance of the *benign* aberrant beats is comparable to a sheep in wolf's clothing. Beware!

## SELECTED READINGS

Gouaux JL, Ashman R: Auricular fibrillation simulating ventricular paroxysmal tachycardia. *Am Heart J* 34:306, 1947.

Marriott HJL Sandler IA: Criteria, old and new, for differentiating between ectopic ventricular beats and aberrant ventricular conduction in the presence of atrial fibrillation. *Prog Cardiovasc Dis* 9:18, 1966.

Nelson WP, Fletcher RD: The "Ashman Phenomenon." *Med Times* 106:96, 1978.

Sandler IA, Marriott HJL: The differential morphology of anomalous ventricular complexes of RBBB-type in lead $V_1$: ventricular ectopy versus aberration. *Circulation* 31:551, 1965.

Sweetwood HM, Boak JG: Aberrant conduction. *Heart and Lung* 6:673, 1977.

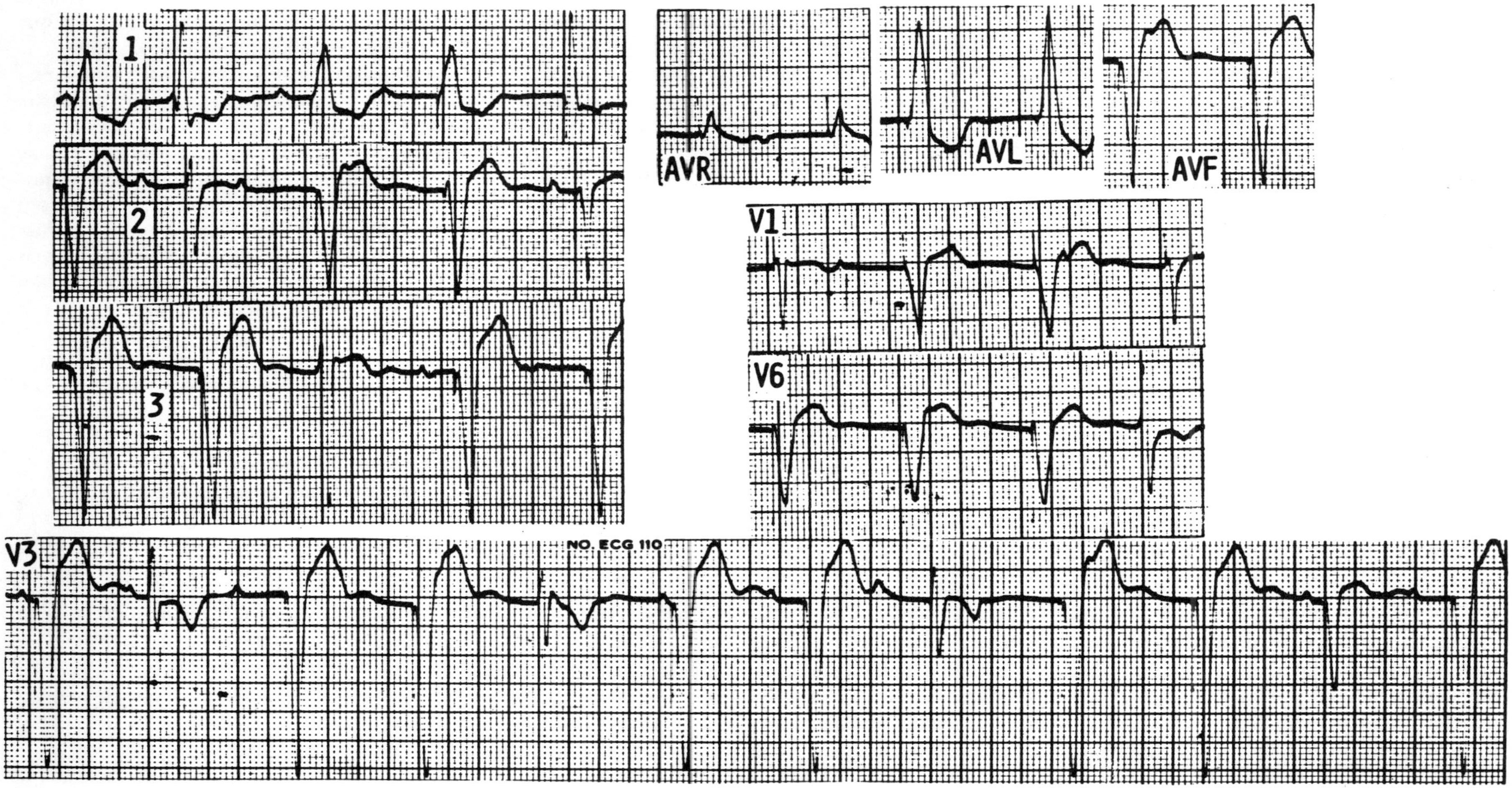


**Figure 20** This tracing is of an 80-year-old woman, hospitalized in heart failure. She was receiving only diuretics.

# NUMBER 20 *Gotcha Under My Skin* Jorge I. Martinez-Lopez

## ELUCIDATION

**Diagnosis**—*Demand-mode artificial pacemaker, functioning normally*

## DISCUSSION

From the tracing presented, numerous conclusions can be arrived at, as discussed briefly below.

An artificial pacemaker is in place. This can be deduced from the visible spikes which precede bizarre QRS complexes, such as seen in the 1st, 3rd, and 4th complexes in bipolar limb leads I and II and in $V_3$. These spikes represent the artifact introduced by the electrical stimulus fired by the pacemaker. Pure, paced beats consist of a spike preceding the corresponding ventricular response.

The amplitude of the spikes indicates the use of a bipolar electrode catheter. Bipolar pacing yields small spikes because both poles are within the paced cardiac chamber. In contrast, with unipolar pacing, one electrode is inside the heart and the other in the body surface; the spikes are large in amplitude and diphasic. Several leads need to be examined because the amplitude may vary from lead to lead, depending upon the spatial orientation of the spike relative to the axis of the lead recorded.

When two consecutive pace beats are present, the firing rate of the pacemaker is 72 per minute.

The morphology of the paced beats in the precordial leads and their spatial orientation in the frontal leads provide information regarding the site of pacing. Classically, right ventricular pacing produces a complete left bundle branch block pattern, or deep and broad S waves in $V_5$ and $V_6$ as seen in the tracing.

Moreover, the abnormal left axis deviation in the frontal leads indicates that pacing occurs at the apex of the right ventricle. Ventricular pacing from the inflow or outflow tract results in a normal axis, while pacing immediately below the pulmonary valve causes right axis or vertical deviation of the mean QRS vector. In contrast, complete right bundle branch block is seen in left ventricular or coronary sinus pacing.

The paced beats are not followed by closely coupled P waves. From this, it can be surmised that there is no retrograde ventriculoatrial conduction.

In some instances, ventricular complexes, though abnormal in duration, are narrower than the paced beats and contain a pacemaker spike. eg, the 4th, 8th, and 11th complexes in $V_3$. When this is observed, two possibilities have to be considered. The first is that these ventricular complexes may represent simultaneous depolarization of the ventricles from the artificial pacemaker and a spontaneous impulse *(true fusion beats)*. In such an event, the duration of the QRS complexes may vary because the two foci do not contribute evenly to ventricular activation. The alternate explanation is that such ventricular complexes may represent *pseudofusion beats;* ie, the spike distorts the QRS complex because of the superimposition of an *ineffectual* spike upon the ventricular complex originating from a spontaneous impulse. Neither of these electrical phenomena indicates malfunction, but constitutes normal function of demand pacemakers.

The pacemaker is in demand mode. This can be rapidly deduced by examining the strip in $V_3$. The second QRS complex is narrower than the paced beats, does not have a spike preceding or buried within it, and represents a spontaneous impulse. The long pause which follows the second ventricular complex is interrupted by a spike (and a captured ventricular complex). It can be concluded that the spontaneous impulse was *sensed* by the pulse generator, and that it was suppressed and reset (recycling without firing) by this beat. Following the spontaneous beat, the pulse generator does not sense any electrophysiologic event within the interval programmed for its escape interval, and fires. Once again, this sequence of events indicates *normal* demand function. One cannot always distinguish between fixed-rate (competitive) and demand pacing in the electrocardiogram unless a natural beat occurs.

Since the interval between the spontaneous beat and the first paced beat is basically equal to the interval between two consecutive spikes, no rate hysteresis is present. Otherwise, the interval between the spontaneous beat and the paced beat would be longer than the interval between two paced beats (automatic interval).

Finally, in many leads P waves are seen occurring regularly at a rate of 79 per minute, and are totally dissociated from both the paced (to be expected) and the spontaneous complexes. The abnormal duration of the spontaneous ventricular complexes indicates an idioventricular rhythm. A diagnosis of complete AV block can be made.

## SELECTED READINGS

Barold SS, Gaidula JJ: Selected electrocardiographic manifestations of cardiac pacing. *Cardiol Digest* July 1972, pp 16–29.

Castellanos A, et al: The electrocardiogram in patients with pacemakers. *Prog Cradiovasc Dis* 13:190–209, 1970.

Castellanos A, Lemberg L: Pacemaker arrhythmias and electrocardiographic recognition of pacemakers. *Circulation* 47:1382–1391, 1973.

## NUMBER 21 *Rhythmic Allotropism* Jorge I. Martinez-Lopez

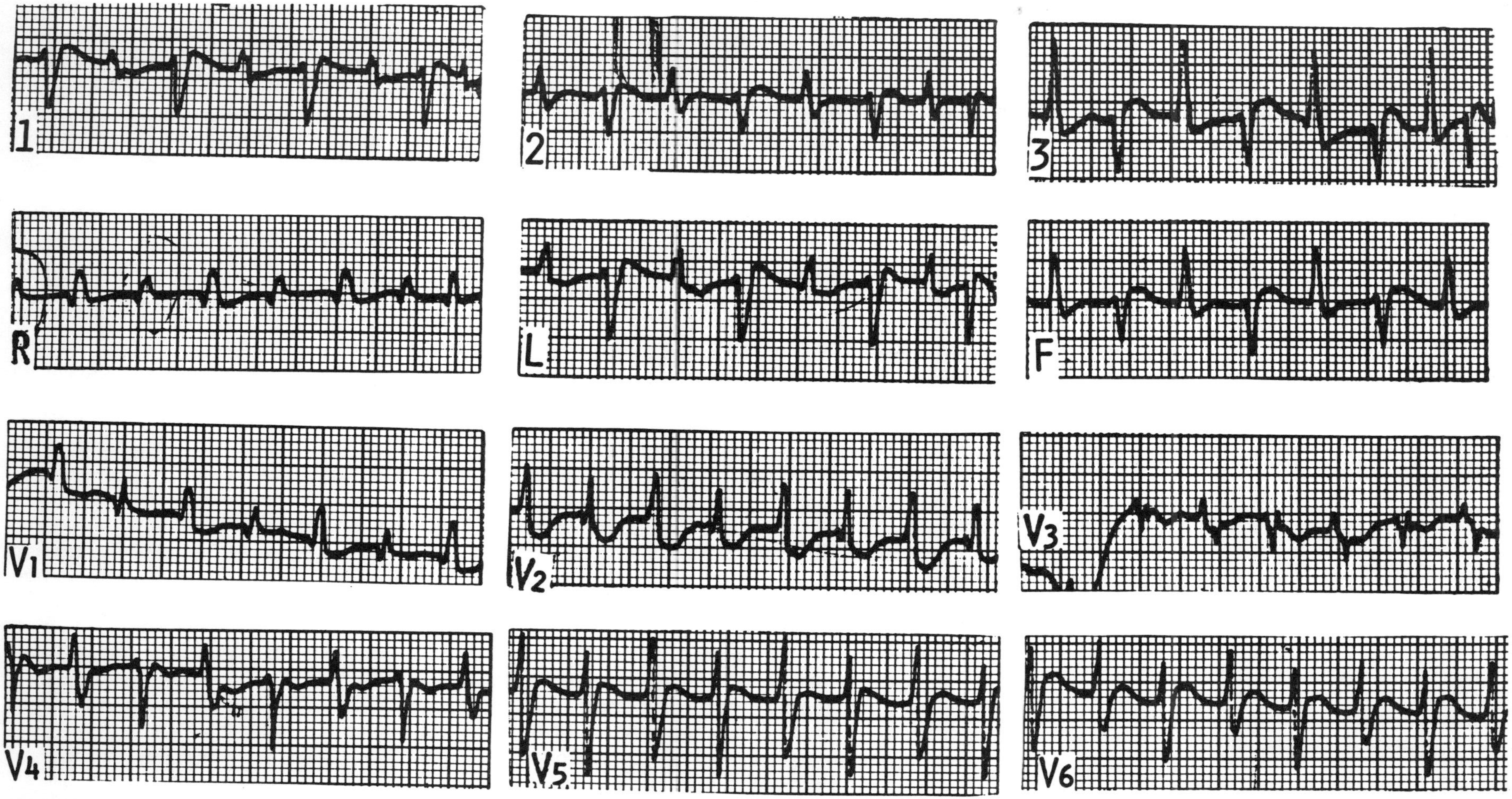


**Figure 21** A 19-year-old primigravida at term was admitted to the obstetrical unit with a diagnosis of "cardiomyopathy." On admission she was found to be in cardiac failure. Nasal oxygen and diuretics were administered. A total of 1.5 mg of digoxin was given intravenously over a period of a few hours. The tracing was recorded after the above measures were instituted.

# NUMBER 21 *Rhythmic Allotropism* Jorge I. Martinez-Lopez

## ELUCIDATION

**Diagnosis**—*Bidirectional tachycardia (BD)*

The tracing shows a relatively regular rhythm, at a rate of 165 per minute. The R-R intervals vary alternately between 0.32 and 0.36 second. One set of QRS complexes is predominantly positive in the limb leads, while the other is negative. In the precordial leads, both sets basically show a right bundle branch block pattern, lasting 0.12 second. No definite P waves are noted.

The arrhythmia was successfully abolished following the administration of several intravenous boluses of diphenylhydantoin sodium.

## DISCUSSION

Bidirectional tachyardia is a rare cardiac arrhythmia. It occurs in a setting of chronic severe heart disease, and is frequently associated with a serious prognosis and a high mortality.

In the majority of patients with the arrhythmia, digitalis has been incriminated as the offending agent. Exceptionally, it has been reported in acute myocardial infarction.

Electrocardiographic recognition of BD usually is not difficult. Ventricular rate is rapid, in the range of 130–180 per minute. Two different ventricular complexes are recorded, alternating rhythmically and, as a rule, but not always, are of opposite polarity. Both ventricular complexes are prolonged in duration and of aberrant configuration. Three variants have been described: a) *type I*—alternating QRS complexes with *equal* diastolic intervals; b) *type II*—alternating QRS complexes with *alternation* of diastolic intervals, ie, alternation of longer and shorter intervals; and c) *type III*—the QRS configurations and the diastolic intervals vary *irregularly*. Type II is the most common. P waves are usually absent.

It may well be that BD is only a descriptive term applicable to a heterogeneous group of cardiac arrhythmias displaying similar electroardiographic configurations. A number of mechanisms have been proposed to explain BD, and some have been confirmed by His bundle electrocardiography. In general, BD has been attributed to: a) a single supraventricular ectopic focus firing rapidly with alternation of conduction down the right and left bundle branches; b) a single or two separate ventricular foci, either with or without circus movements; c) two ectopic foci, one supraventricular and the other ventricular in origin; and d) a persistent junctional rhythm with premature ventricular contractions in bigeminy. In any given case, the surface electrocardiogram may not provide the necessary data to determine which specific electrophysiologic phenomenon is in operation.

There is no universally successful single form of treatment. If digitalis is implicated as the inciting agent, it must be discontinued and measures to counteract its effect instituted.

## SELECTED READINGS


Cohen SI, Deisseroth A, Hecht HS: Infra-His bundle origin of bidirectional tachycardia. *Circulation* 48:32, 1973.

Rosenbaum MB, Elizari MV, Lazzari JO: The mechanism of bidirectional tachycardia. *Am Heart J* 78:4, 1969.

Scherf D, Kisch B: Ventricular tachycardia with variform ventricular complexes. *Bull NY Med Coll* 2:73, 1939.

## NUMBER 22 *Foxy Lad* Jorge I. Martinez-Lopez

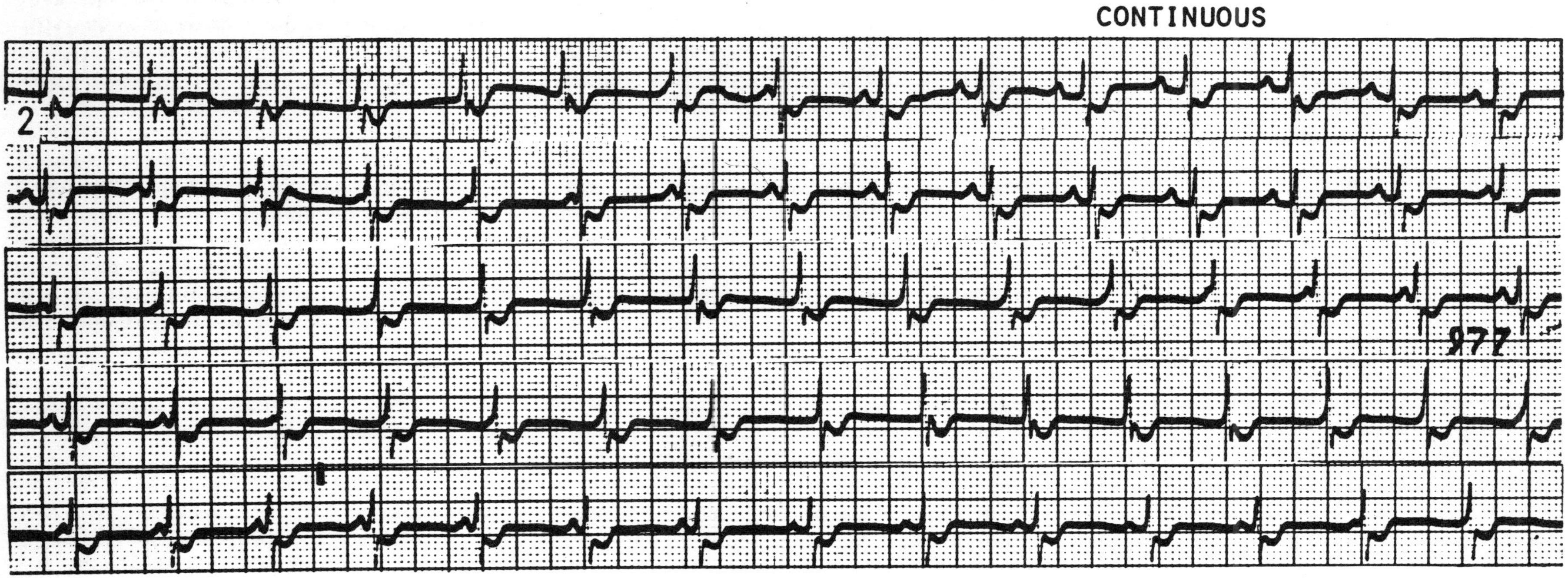


**Figure 22** The tracing is of a 17-year-old male, taken on admission 18 hours after ingesting an undisclosed number of tablets for suicidal purposes.

## NUMBER 22 *Foxy Lad* Jorge I. Martinez-Lopez

### ELUCIDATION

**Diagnosis**—*AV dissociation due to massive digitalis intoxication*

The cardiac rate is regular at about 100 times per minute. The configuration of the QRS complexes indicates normal intraventricular conduction. The prominent feature of this tracing is the constant movement, back and forth, of the P waves. At times, they are in front of, sometimes behind, or concealed within, the ventricular complexes. The atrial and ventricular rates are essentially similar though dissociated (isorhythmic AV dissociation), due to enhancement of a junctional subsidiary focus with resulting junctional tachycardia.

This youngster attempted suicide by ingesting a large number of digitalis leaf tablets belonging to his grandfather. His stay in the hospital was uncomplicated other than for cardiac arrhythmias, which included AV dissociation, followed by first degree AV block before normal sinus rhythm returned spontaneously. Management consisted of intravenous administration of fluids, electrocardiographic monitoring, and pervenous insertion of a temporary demand pacemaker. He recovered.

### DISCUSSION

Digitalis or *foxglove* has been in clinical use for nearly 200 years. Despite its wide usage and beneficial therapeutic effects, toxicity is a frequent complication. Digitalis intoxication may occur in two major clinical settings. The commonest form results from either relative or absolute excesses secondary to chronic administration of digitalis in patients with cardiac disease (iatrogenic). Signs of toxicity generally appear at plasma levels above 2 ng/ml for digoxin or 20 ng/ml for digitoxin.

In contrast, deliberate intoxication is infrequently observed and results from ingestion (or injection) of large amounts of digitalis either accidentally or as a suicidal gesture. Under these circumstances, plasma levels rise more acutely and are higher than during chronic administration of the drug. In the majority of reports, digitoxin, digoxin, and lanatoside C were used. Rarely has digitalis leaf been used.

In both forms of intoxication, the presenting manifestations are cardiac and/or extracardiac. However, the presence or absence of underlying cardiac disease appears to modify the observed cardiac disturbances in massive digitalis intoxication. Whereas a variety of ventricular ectopic rhythms is frequent in those with cardiac disease, *ventricular arrhythmias are absent in patients with no evidence of heart disease.* In this last group of patients, rhythm disturbances most frequently seen include atrial premature beats and development of sinoatrial or AV block.

A serious and relatively frequent complication of massive digitalis intoxication is hyperkalemia. Presumably, the primary mechanism for this potentially lethal complication is inhibition of the sodium—potassium pump, leading to hyperpolarization of cardiac cells and to ventricular standstill. Hyperkalemia may also be due partly to the frequently associated oliguria secondary to systemic hypotension.

A number of factors determine the eventual outcome of massive digitalis intoxication. Those having an adverse effect on prognosis include older age, presence of heart disease or chronic pulmonary disease, hyperkalemia, renal or hepatic insufficiency, and "myocardial irritability."

Accidental or suicidal digitalis intoxication can be successfully managed in most cases by appropriate use of antiarrhythmic drugs and vagolytic drugs combined, when necessary, with temporary pervenous pacing. Management requires immediate hospitalization, preferably in the MICU or CCU, with continuous electrocardiographic monitoring so as to discover and treat potentially lethal arrhythmias; clinical observations and continuous electrocardiographic monitoring are better guides to prognosis and choice of therapy than are determinations of blood concentrations of digitalis.

A final word on potassium. Crucial to the management of the acutely intoxicated patient are serial measurements of serum potassium levels. Obviously, in the presence of hyperkalemia, supplemental potassium may prove lethal to the patient. Accordingly, supplemental potassium should not be used as a matter of routine without due consideration of the type of rhythm disturbance, serum potassium level, and renal function. Very high serum levels may require dialysis which, of course, is useless in eliminating digitalis. Severe hyperkalemia may prove refractory to treatment, including the failure to elicit a ventricular response with pacing.

## SELECTED READINGS

Asplund J, Edhag O, et al: Four cases of massive digitalis poisoning. *Acta Med Scand* 189:239–297, 1971.

Bertler A, Gustafson A, Redfors A: Massive digoxin intoxication. *Acta Med Scand* 194:245–249, 1973.

Smith TW, Willerson JT: Suicidal and accidental digoxin ingestion. *Circulation* 44: 29–36, 1971.

# NUMBER 23 *Rebel Without a Pause* Jorge I. Martinez-Lopez

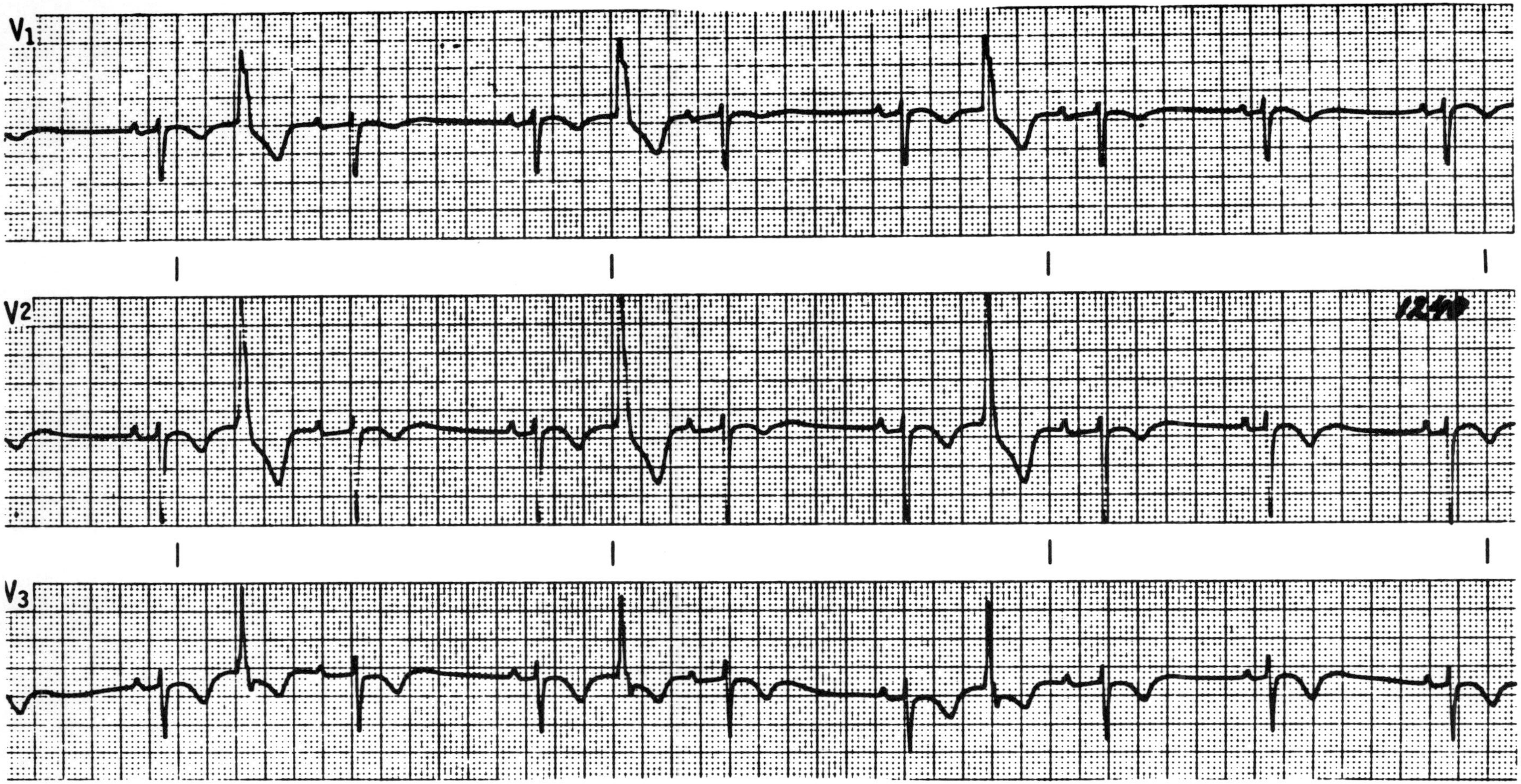


**Figure 23** The tracings are of a 57-year-old woman with coronary artery disease manifested by angina pectoris. She was taking coronary vasodilators.

## ELUCIDATION

**Diagnosis**—*Ventricular premature beats with concealed retrograde conduction*

Sinus bradycardia with normal intraventricular conduction is present. T waves are inverted in all three leads.

Prominently visible are the wide and aberrant QRS complexes of opposite polarity, which represent ventricular premature beats. These ventricular complexes are "sandwiched" between two consecutive sinus beats and do not disturb the P-P intervals. The P-R interval of the sinus beat preceding the ectopic beat measures 0.18 sec. That this prolongation in the P-R interval is related to the ectopic beat can be established by noticing the stable P-R interval in the last two sinus beats. Accordingly, concealed retrograde conduction of the ventricular ectopic impulse into the junctional area can be deduced.

## DISCUSSION

Ventricular premature beats (VPB) are common in the clinical practice of medicine and represent ectopic activity that precedes the expected discharge of the basic rhythm. They can occur in the presence or absence of heart disease, and may or may not be associated with symptoms.

The typical VPB are: a) abnormal in duration and configuration; b) accompanied by ST-T wave changes; c) not preceded by a premature P wave; d) followed by a full compensatory pause; and e) bear a constant temporal relationship to the preceding beat of the dominant rhythm, termed *"fixed coupling."*

Although most VPB exceed 0.11 sec, some are narrow and are presumed to originate within high fascicular or divisional segments of the conduction system. Even when broad and bizarre, the configuration of VPB may also vary depending upon the ventricular chamber (right or left), and the specific area within the ventricle (posterior or anterior wall, base or apex, right or left septal surface) from which they originate. In a given patient, the origin of VPB may be unifocal or multifocal.

As mentioned earlier, VPB are most often followed by a full compensatory pause because they do *not* disturb the sinus rhythm. In other words, following the VPB, the oncoming normally discharged sinus impulse encounters refractoriness downgrade in the wake of the VPB and cannot depolarize the ventricles, ie, it is physiologically blocked distally. Since the sinus rhythm is not disturbed, the SA node fires subsequently at the expected time. The full compensatory pause represents the interval from the conducted beat before the VPB to the conducted beat following the VPB, and is equal to two normal sinus cycles. The "blocked" P wave can usually be identified in the ST segment or T wave of the VPB and has to be differentiated from P waves caused by retrograde entry of the ventricular impulse into the atria.

Less frequently, VPB may take exception to the rules and behave in several ways. To understand these exceptions it is essential to appreciate that the conducting system of the heart allows bidirectional traffic of electrical impulses, ie, anterograde and retrograde. Accordingly, impulses originating within the ventricles, under the proper set of circumstances, can enter the conducting system, travel variable distances in a ventriculoatrial direction, and affect subsequent electrophysiologic events. Retrograde penetration may be manifest or concealed, and result in pauses which are either "incomplete," absent, or longer than a full compensatory pause, or in reciprocal ventricular extrasystoles (echo beats).

Incomplete compensatory pauses occur when the ventricular ectopic impulse travels retrograde into the atria, discharges, and resets the SA node. In this situation, the interval from the conducted beat before the VPB to the conducted beat following the VPB is *less* than two normal sinus cycles. Alternatively, such retrograde discharge may cause abnormal suppression of the SA node, and results in an interval *longer* than two sinus cycles. A last possibility is that the ventricular impulse, upon reaching the atria or AV node, may turn around and return downgrade to or toward its area of origin (reentry), causing a reciprocal ventricular extrasystole.

The tracing presented here displays VPB which are "sandwiched" between two consecutive sinus beats and are *not* followed by a compensatory pause (interpolated). More important is the observed lengthening of the P-R interval following the VPB, when compared to the one preceding it. This can be attributed to *concealed* retrograde conduction. This means that the VPB journeyed retrogradely along the conducting system, was unsuccessful in reaching the atria, but reached the AV junction where it left a wake of refractoriness. The next sinus impulse forms and emerges from the SA node at the expected time and travels antegrade but, as a result of the concealed conduction by the VPB, it is slowed down through the junctional area, and the P-R interval is prolonged. Less frequently, interpolated ventricular bigeminy with concealed retrograde conduction into the AV node may lengthen successive P-R intervals progressively until an atrial impulse is dropped, producing retrograde Wenckebach periodicity.

In summary, do not rely on the full compensatory pause to make a diagnosis of VPB. Some are rebels without a pause!

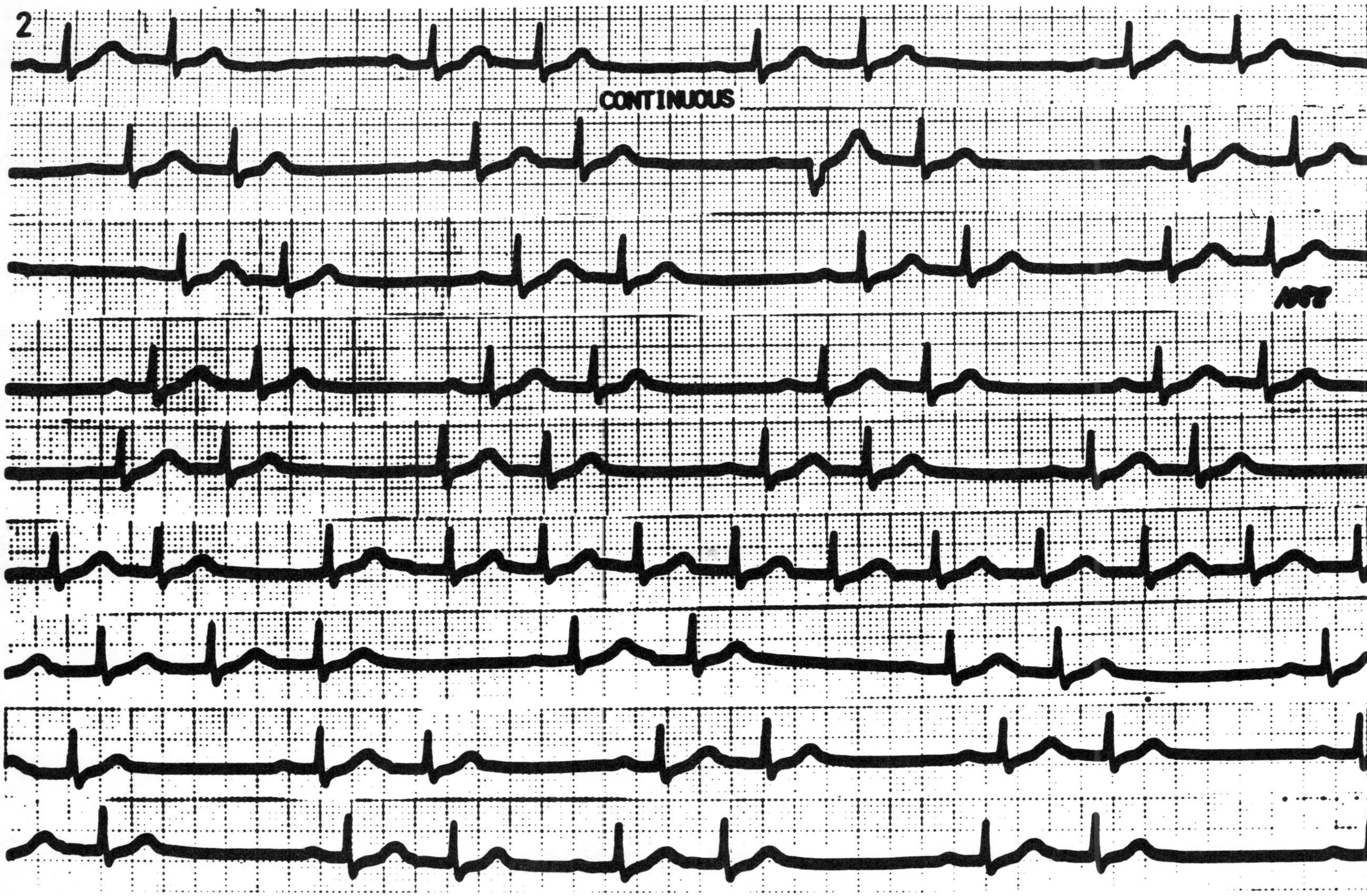


**Figure 24** The tracing was taken on a 75-year-old man with repeated episodes of near-fainting attributed to transient cerebral attacks.

## NUMBER 24 *A Sinus Condition* Jorge I. Martinez-Lopez

### ELUCIDATION

**Diagnosis**—*Sick sinus syndrome*

The basic mechanism is sinus in nature. First degree AV block (P-R interval, 0.22 sec) and normal intraventricular conduction (narrow QRS) are present.

Sinus rhythm is associated with atrial premature beats in bigeminy in the major portion of the tracing. These beats have a long P′-R interval. The ectopic P wave is seen deforming the downstroke of the T wave, with slight variation of the coupling interval. Pauses following the premature beats are excessively long. From this, one may conclude that the sinus node has been reset by the ectopic impulse, resulting in abnormal suppression.

The fifth QRS complex in the second row represents a ventricular escape beat. The P wave in front of it occurs fortuitously and is not conducted. It is blocked by the refractoriness encountered downgrade in the wake of the ventricular escape beat. An atrial premature beat follows the escape beat, but it is conducted in the same manner as previous premature beats (long P′-R interval and narrow QRS). This association discards the possibility that earlier and subsequent couplets represent reciprocal beats. This is important because the faster rhythm seen in the sixth row raises the question of re-entrant tachycardia. In view of the above, it appears likely that the faster rhythm observed is due to enhanced automaticity in the atrial ectopic centers, for whatever reasons.

### DISCUSSION

The sinoatrial node (SAN) is a small structure composed of highly specialized cells, located at the junction of the superior vena cava and the right atrium. Centrally located in the SAN is its artery, which originates from the proximal portion of either the right or the left circumflex coronary artery. In its periphery, the SAN, although in close proximity to the atrial pericardium, is entirely surrounded by an anatomic barrier, the perinodal buffer zone, through which electrical activity must pass on its way out of or into the SAN.

Of all the components of the conducting system possessing inherent automaticity, it is the dominant pacemaker of the heart. Electrical impulses develop spontaneously within the SAN, presumably in the P cells, at rates ranging from 60 to 100 times per minute in adults. Rates are much faster in children, but gradually slow down with advancing age. Recognized normal variants of impulse formation are sinus bradycardia, sinus tachycardia, and sinus arrhythmia.

Normal function of the SAN can be modified by a variety of extrinsic and intrinsic factors, as well as by the interaction between these two major determinants. Hence, sinus node dysfunction may result from alteration in one or more of these loci, and is expressed clinically as either disturbances in impulse formation, in impulse conduction, or both.

The term "sick sinus syndrome" (SSS), first introduced by Lown, was popularized and expanded by Ferrer to characterize sinus node dysfunction in the clinical setting. Accordingly, it is *not* a diagnosis, but rather a descriptive and collective name given to a wide variety of chronic episodic or sustained malfunctions of the SAN in the presence or absence of clinically recognizable heart disease. Use of the term is not applicable when the observed malfunction is the result of drug administration.

In general, SSS is seen twice as often in females as in males. Its incidence peaks at about age 70, but it may be seen in young persons following the Mustard procedure for complete transposition of the great vessels, and also as a familial syndrome.

Clinical manifestations vary widely and are not specific for the disorder. They are determined by the type of sinus dysfunction, by the resulting hemodynamic alterations, and by the underlying status of the heart and of the central and coronary circulations. The most common symptoms are dizziness, syncope, cardiac failure, and angina pectoris.

The electrocardiographic features of SSS include: a) pauses in sinus rhythm caused by sinus arrest, third-degree SA block, or repetitive concealed sinus exit block; b) periods of second-degree SA block; c) episodes of alternating sinus bradycardia and rapid atrial arrhythmias, the so-called "bradycardia-tachycardia syndrome" (BTS); d) persistent, severe, and unexplained symptomatic sinus bradycardia; e) chronic atrial fibrillation with a slow ventricular response *not due to medica-*

*tions,* and e) inability to resume stable sinus rhythm following electrical cardioversion.

Frequently, however, the patient afflicted with SSS may not exhibit any of the above ECG features when seen by the physician because of their episodic recurrence. In such cases, it is desirable to resort to Holter monitoring to validate the presence of sinus dysfunction.

In patients presenting with slow sinus rates, blunted response of the SAN may be verified by the use of isotonic or isometric exercise tests, by pharmacologic interventions, such as intravenous administration of isoproterenol or atropine, and by other bedside maneuvers.

More recently, invasive electrophysiologic studies have added new dimensions in the assessment of patients suspected of having SSS. They are carried out in the cardiac catheterization laboratory, and include extrastimulus methods and oversuppression by rapid atrial pacing. Utilizing these procedures, measurements can be made of the sinus-to-atrial conduction time (SACT), sinoatrial recovery time, both uncorrected (SANRT) and corrected ($SANRT_C$), and intrinsic heart rate (IHR). In addition, His bundle electrocardiography is performed concurrently because abnormal conduction and refractory periods are found within the specialized AV-His-Purkinje system in about two-thirds of these patients.

Once the diagnosis of the SSS has been confirmed, how is the patient managed? Long-term medical management is frequently unsuccessful because of unresponsiveness to pharmacologic agents, their short duration of action, and intolerable side effects. Hence, virtually every patient with SSS requires implantation of a permanent pacemaker, either ventricular demand-mode or AV sequential. Atrial pacemakers are seldom used because of the associated conduction disturbances at the AV node itself or in the His-Purkinje system, and because of the potential for further depression of abnormal sinus function by the implanted pacemaker.

A special problem is posed by patients with BTS. Antiarrhythmic drugs may control tachyarrhythmias, but they often impair conduction in the AV node-His-Purkinje system. For this reason, it is often necessary to combine cardiac pacing with antiarrhythmic drugs.

Despite optimal management of patients with SSS, the long-term prognosis is not favorable. The great majority of deaths are cardiac-related.

## SELECTED READINGS

Ferrer MI: The sick sinus syndrome. *Circulation* 47:635–641, 1973.

Goldreyer BN: Sinus node dysfunction—a physiologic consideration of arrhythmias involving the sinus node. *Cardiovasc Clin* 6:180–198, 1974.

Mandel WJ, et al: Assessment of sinus node function in patients with the sick sinus syndrome. *Circulation* 46:761–769, 1972.

Moss AJ, Davis RJ: Brady-tachy syndrome. *Prog Cardiovasc Dis* 16:439–454, 1974.

Rubenstein JJ, et al: Clinical spectrum of the sick sinus syndrome. *Circulation* 46:5–13, 1972.

## NUMBER 25 *Premature, Immature, or Postmature?* Jorge I. Martinez-Lopez

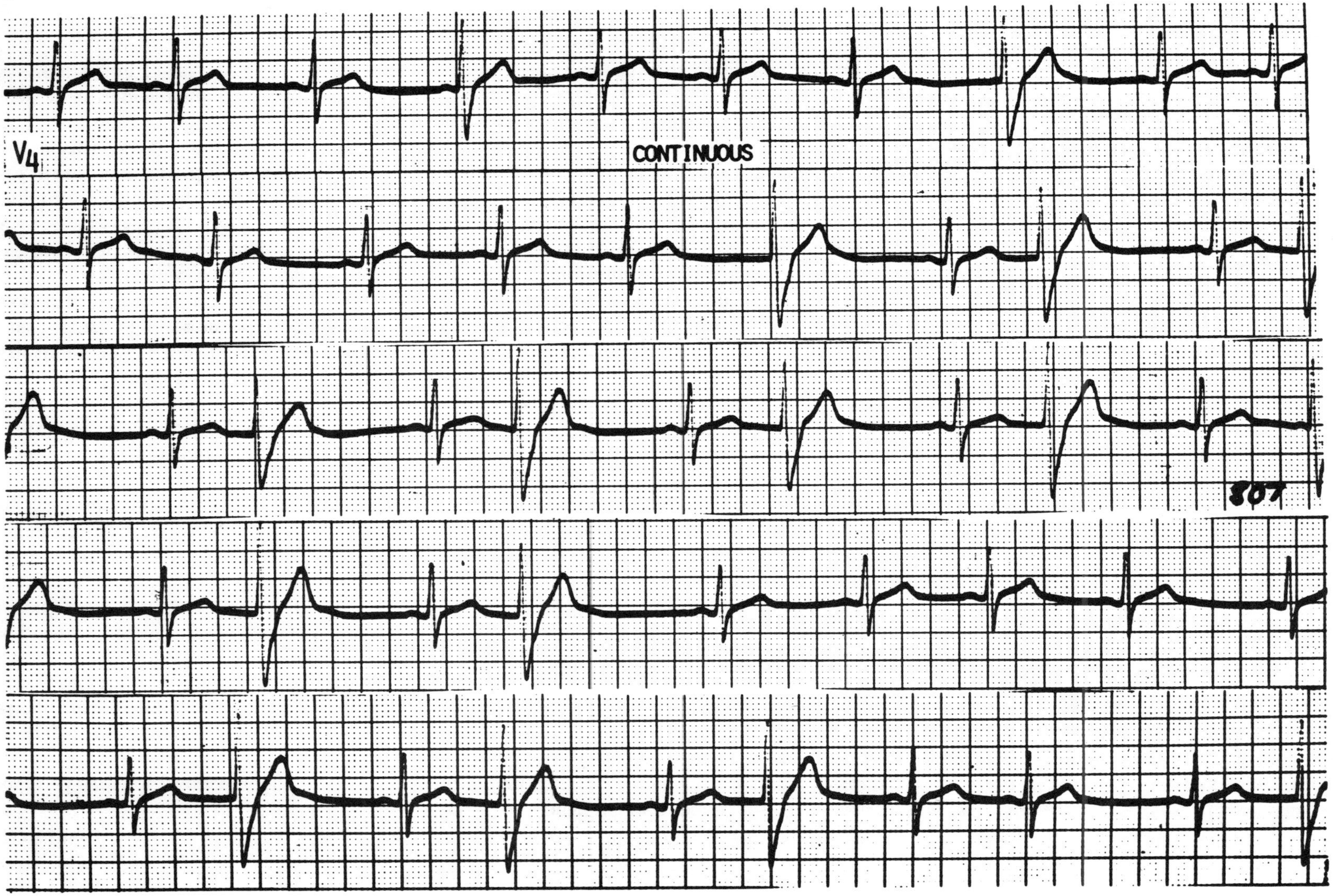


**Figure 25** The tracing is of a 34-year-old man admitted to the hospital for open reduction of a fractured wrist. There was no previous history of heart disease. He was on no medications.

# NUMBER 25 *Premature, Immature, or Postmature?* Jorge I. Martinez-Lopez

## ELUCIDATION

**Diagnosis**—*Ventricular parasystole*

The basic rhythm is sinus in origin in association with sinus arrhythmia. The PR, QRS, and QT intervals of the normally conducted beats are normal in duration.

The prominent finding in this tracing is the intermittent appearance of QRS complexes of abnormal duration (0.12 sec). The morphology of all of the complexes is similar, suggesting a single focus of origin within the ventricles. The coupling intervals between the sinus beats and the ventricular ectopic beats vary widely. Some ectopic beats occur late in diastole ("postmature"), while others occur in early ("premature") or mid-diastole ("immature"). Therefore, these complexes do *not* represent escape beats or ventricular premature beats!

A last feature of the abnormal ventricular complexes is their recurrence with predictable regularity. Consecutive ectopic beats containing an intervening sinus beat display intervals varying between 1840 and 1880 msec. In contrast, long intervals containing two or more intervening sinus beats are close multiples of the shorter intervals. No fusion beats are present.

Based on these observations, the interpreter can confidently establish the diagnosis of *classic* ventricular parasystole.

## DISCUSSION

The presence of one or more abnormally prolonged QRS complexes (0.12 second or longer) on the ECG should prompt the physician to consider two possibilities: abnormal conduction of a supraventricular impulse (aberration, bundle branch block or pre-excitation) versus ventricular ectopy. Ventricular ectopic rhythms include: premature beats, accelerated idioventricular rhythm, escape beats, parasystole, tachycardia, flutter, and fibrillation.

*Parasystole* is an uncommon arrhythmia occasionally observed in healthy subjects but more frequently in a variety of clinical disorders. No evidence has been presented that it is drug-induced or related to electrolyte levels. Parasystole can occur anywhere in the heart, but it is most frequently ventricular, less commonly junctional, and rarely atrial. The discussion which follows is limited to classic ventricular parasystole.

Ventricular parasystole frequently goes unrecognized for two major reasons. First, many physicians are not familiar with it and casually dismiss the ectopic beats as premature beats. Second, the usual 12-lead tracing is not of sufficient length to raise the index of suspicion. For this reason, rhythm strips should be obtained whenever ectopic beats are present.

Before describing the features in the ECG, it is essential to discuss briefly the concept of parasystole. In ventricular parasystole, an area within the ventricle (in the distal specialized conduction system) secedes from the surrounding myocardium and becomes a *parasystolic focus.* In proclaiming its independence from the basic driving mechanism, it acquires enhanced automaticity, firing regularly and asynchronously, and competes with the prevailing rhythm—with which it coexists—to activate the ventricles. Hence, the ventricles can be depolarized dually by two fronts: by the predominant rhythm and by the parasystolic focus.

For the parasystolic focus to survive and coexist with the basic rhythm, it must shield itself from oncoming impulses. Otherwise, the parasystolic focus would be penetrated and discharged. This is referred to as *protection* or *entrance* block. This self-generated protection, however, is a two-edged sword for it also creates a physiologic barrier which impedes emergence of the impulse from within the parasystolic focus; this is termed *exit block.* The degree of *entrance* and *exit blocks* may be complete or incomplete and may vary in the same patient.

The electrophysiologic characteristics of the parasystolic focus mentioned above provide the simplest electrocardiographic clue with which to suspect ventricular parasystole: the recurrence of ectopic beats coupled at widely varying intervals to beats of the predominant rhythm. Some occur early in diastole, others in mid-diastole, and still others in late diastole. In contrast, virtually all true unifocal ventricular premature beats display fixed coupling intervals, because they are "forced beats" resulting from reentrant phenomena.

Once parasystole is suspected by the variability of the coupling intervals, the diagnosis can be established by careful analysis of long rhythm strips, which includes measuring the interectopic intervals and searching for fusion beats.

Two different interectopic intervals are recognized and are related to the inherent rate of discharge of the parasystolic focus and to the degree of exit block present. The first is the *shortest* interectopic interval. It is the measurable interval between two successive parasystolic beats *without* an intervening beat from the basic rhythm. From this interval, the inherent rate of the parasystolic focus can be deduced. *Longer* interectopic intervals, the second type, are those between two parasystolic beats *containing* intervening beats from the basic rhythm. These intervals reflect the degree of exit block and should be close multiples of the shortest interectopic interval; precisely constant interectopic intervals are extremely rare.

From the above, it should be clear that the *parasystolic* and the *manifest* rates are seldom equal. The first represents the inherent firing rate of the parasystolic focus, while the latter reflects the degree of exit block. In other words, the manifest rate is determined by the number of impulses originating in the parasystolic focus which are successful in emerging and discharging the surrounding myocardium. Because of the exit block, this number is usually less than that of the intrinsic rate and is expressed as a ratio (2:1, etc).

Fusion beats are very common in ventricular parasystole but their presence is *not* essential to the diagnosis. They represent simultaneous or nearly simultaneous activation of the ventricles by impulses coming from different directions. The net result is a ventricular complex that is "intermediate in form between the pure complexes resulting from the differently originating excitation waves."

Why should the physician be aware of ventricular parasystole? In the first place, because it is a *benign* arrhythmia. Having no important effects in hemodynamics, it does not produce cardiac symptoms nor does it affect mortality; secondly, because it is *not* a manifestation of digitalis intoxication or electrolyte abnormalities; lastly, because it is *not* a forerunner of more serious arrhythmias, such as ventricular tachycardia and ventricular fibrillation. Its existence, therefore, should not elicit the "lidocaine bolus reflex!"

## SELECTED READINGS

Chung EKY: Parasystole. *Prog Cardiovasc Dis* 11:64–81, 1968.

Pick A, Langendorf R: Parasystole and its variants. *Med Clin North Am* 60:125–147, 1976.

Watanabe Y: Reassessment of parasystole. *Am Heart J* 81:451–466, 1971.

## NUMBER 26 *A Lot of Non-Sense* Jorge I. Martinez-Lopez

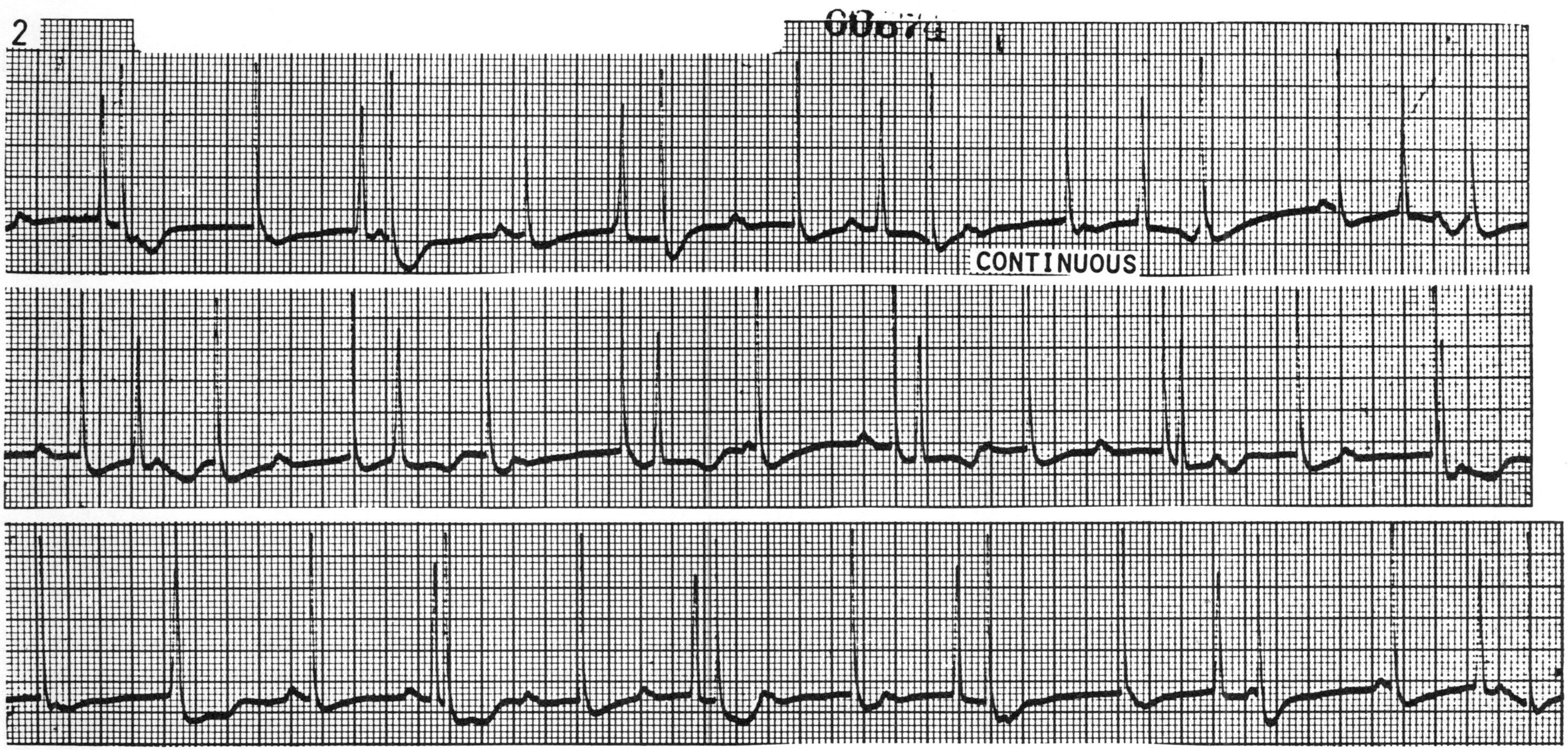


**Figure 26** This tracing was taken on a 69-year-old woman in the outpatient clinic. She was a long-standing hypertensive with repeated episodes of cardiac failure. Medications included methyldopa, hydrochlorothiazide, and digoxin.

## NUMBER 26 *A Lot of Non-Sense* Jorge I. Martinez-Lopez

### ELUCIDATION

**Diagnosis**—*Pacemaker dysfunction, and complete AV block with junctional mechanism*

Careful analysis of the tracing reveals three prominent features: a) an atrial rate of 84 per minute; b) a slow ventricular rate, approximately 42 per minute, with QRS complexes of normal duration—junctional—having no temporal relationship to the atrial impulses; and c) pacemaker artifacts occurring regularly at 72 times per minute, neither sensing natural beats nor capturing ventricular musculature, and "marching through" the atrial and ventricular complexes. This last feature facilitates the diagnosis of *pacemaker dysfunction.*

### DISCUSSION

The electrocardiogram is the single most important tool in evaluating pacemaker function. Understanding the basic principles of pacemaking is essential in order to make an accurate assessment. Lack of knowledge often results in an erroneous diagnosis of pacemaker dysfunction. This error is compounded when it leads to unnecessary explantation and reimplantation of a new pacemaker, with the attendant risks to the patient and the expenses incurred.

Artificial pacemakers, whether temporary or permanent, consist of three major components: the electrical generator, the catheter, and the electrode (or electrodes) attached to the catheter. The electrical impulse generated reaches the terminal electrode via the length of the catheter and, when in contact with myocardium, depolarizes it, causing cardiac contraction. Fault in one or more of the components or lack of contact with myocardium results in pacemaker dysfunction.

The majority of problems encountered during cardiac pacemaking are related to: a) stimulus release; b) stimulation or capture; and c) sensing.

In the tracing shown here, the electrical stimulus *was released* regularly at a fixed rate as shown by the regularly recurring pacemaker spikes. Hence, the generator was not at fault.

Secondly, the recording shows that the released stimulus *failed to capture* or depolarize the recipient chamber, in this case, the right ventricle.

Lastly, since the pacemaker spike recurred constantly and regularly, it can be concluded that the implanted demand pacemaker *was not sensing* the natural beats and was behaving in the fixed-rate mode. In that context, the generator was performing well, ie, as a *demand pacemaker.* In other words, since it did not sense any electrical activity during the pre-set interval, it escaped at a regular rate, the so-called *automatic interval,* even though it failed to capture the right ventricle.

What is a physician to do? The combination of non-sense and no captures should prompt the physician to consider an improperly positioned or "floating" catheter. Cardiac fluoroscopy on the patient presented here showed the catheter to be lying freely in the right atrial chamber. Repositioning the catheter resulted in right ventricular capture, with a 1:1 pacemaker-to-ventricular response.

### SELECTED READINGS

Castellanos A Jr, et al: Cardiac pacemakers. *Cardiovasc Clin* 3:31, 1971.

Furman S: Cardiac pacing and pacemakers. VI. Analysis of pacemaker malfunction. *Am Heart J* 94:378–386, 1977.

Lown B, Kosowsky BD: Artificial cardiac pacemakers. *N Engl J Med* 283:907–916, 971–977, 1012–1031, 1970.

# NUMBER 27 *A Matter of Position* Jorge I. Martinez-Lopez

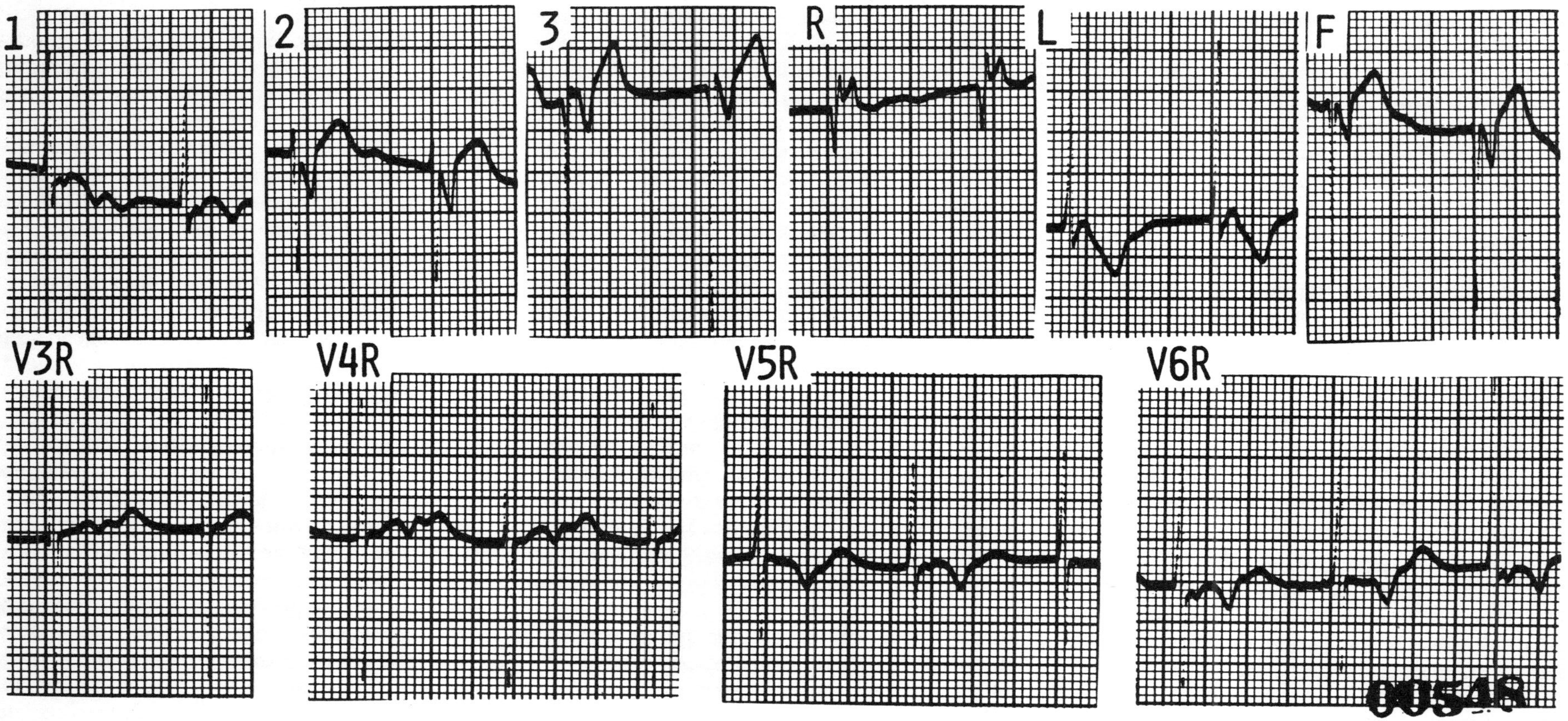


**Figure 27** The tracing is of a 2-year-old girl hospitalized for cardiac evaluation. She was on no medications.

## NUMBER 27 *A Matter of Position* Jorge I. Martinez-Lopez

### ELUCIDATION

**Diagnosis**—*Junctional rhythm and dextrocardia*

The rate is 107/min and regular. Inverted P waves follow the QRS complexes in leads II, III, $aV_F$, and $V_4$–$V_6$; they are upright in the remaining leads. The R-P′ interval is short. The QRS complexes are narrow, indicating that an ectopic supraventricular *(junctional)* focus controls ventricular response. The reversed polarity of the P waves which follow the ventricular complexes results from retrograde activation of the atrial musculature by the same junctional pacemaker. There is no reentry of the atrial front.

Further analysis of the QRS complexes, particularly those in the precordial leads, is thought-provoking! In the chest leads, the prominent feature is the rapidly progressive loss of the R waves and amplitude of the QRS complexes as the electrode moves from right to left. Once this is noted, a second glance at the frontal leads leads one to conclude that I is recorded upside down, and that leads II and III, and $aV_R$ and $aV_L$ are reversed, respectively. From this analysis, it is simple to arrive at a diagnosis of *dextrocardia.*

### DISCUSSION

*Dextrocardia* is the commonest cardiac malposition. Others include dextroversion, mesocardia and mesoversion, levoversion, and *abnormal* levocardia (since levocardia is the normal position of the heart in the chest). Any one of these may occur with normal or abnormal visceral situs (situs solitus or situs inversus), with normal or abnormally related great arteries (normal or transposed), and may or may not be associated with other congenital anomalies or acquired cardiac disorders. This discussion is limited to the "mirror-image" dextrocardia (classic dextrocardia).

Classic dextrocardia is the least complicated of all cardiac malpositions, seldom being associated with other malformations or with shortened life span. It is characterized by *situs inversus* (greater lobe of the liver, ventral atrium, and the suprahepatic segment of the inverior vena cava are on the left). The heart is in the right hemithorax, with the apex directed also toward the right.

Stimulus impulse formation is initiated normally in the sinoatrial node, but now progresses from left to right from the venous to the arterial atrium, and downgrade across the AV node, into the arterial ventricle and then into the venous ventricle. Hence, when the electrocardiogram is recorded conventionally, the reversed spatial alignment of the cardiac chambers and specialized conduction system of the heart introduces alterations in the appearance and contour of the atrial and ventricular complexes.

In the presence of sinus mechanisms, the following findings in the conventional electrocardiogram are consistent with, and should alert the interpreter to consider, the diagnosis of classic dextrocardia:

a. The P vector is directed rightward, inferiorly, and slightly anteriorly. Accordingly, P waves are inverted in leads I and $aV_L$, positive in leads II, III, $aV_R$ and $aV_F$, and change from positive to negative from right to left precordial leads.

b. The QRS complex is inverted in lead I and, in the precordial leads, shows a progressive loss of R wave from right to left.

c. The T wave is upside down in lead I and upright in $aV_R$.

It must be emphasized that some of these electrocardiographic alterations may be produced when the recorder (technician, student, or physician) inadvertently attaches the right arm wire electrode to the left arm and vice versa ("technical dextrocardia"). In such instances, the frontal leads are similar to and mimic classic dextrocardia: lead I is recorded upside down, lead II is actually lead III, III is II, $aV_R$ is $aV_L$, and $aV_L$ is $aV_R$. Once recorded, it may not be possible to determine the locations of the lead wires. Two further observations readily assist in eliminating the possibility of classic dextrocardia: a) P waves remain upright in the left precordial leads during sinus rhythms, and b) the expected transition in the QRS complexes over the precordial leads is retained.

In right-sided hearts, a frequent problem is whether dextroversion or classic dextrocardia is present. In contrast to the latter, the atria preserve their usual relationship in the frontal plane, and the left ventricle lies *anterior* to the right in dextroversion. Accordingly, P waves are upright in lead I in dextroversion in sinus rhythm. Moreover, careful analysis of the precordial leads makes possible the precise determination of the relative position of the two ventricles in patients with a right-sided heart.

The conventional tracing presented here showed the expected changes of dextrocardia in the ventricular complexes. However, analysis of the location and polarity of the atrial complexes indicated retrograde activation of the atria from the junctional pacemaker site. In addition, the "corrected" tracing taken subsequently (not shown here) also displayed abnormal left axis deviation and abnormally high amplitude of the ventricular complexes over the right chest.

A "corrected" tracing may be obtained simply by reversing the position of the right and left arm wire electrodes, and by recording the precordial leads using the conventional $V_2$ as $V_1$, and proceeding from left to right with $V_{2_R}$, $V_{3_R}$ etc.

## SELECTED READINGS

Anselmi G, et al: Systematization and clinical study of dextroversion, mirror-image dextrocardia, and laevoversion. *Br Heart J* 34:1085–1098, 1972.

Daves ML, Pryor R: Cardiac positions. *Am Heart J* 79:408–421, 1970.

Mirowski M, et al: Negative P waves in lead I in dextroversion: differential diagnosis from mirror-image dextrocardia. *Circulation* 26:413–420, 1962.

Van Praagh R, et al: Diagnosis of the anatomic types of congenital dextrocardia. *Am J Cardiol* 15:234–247, 1965.

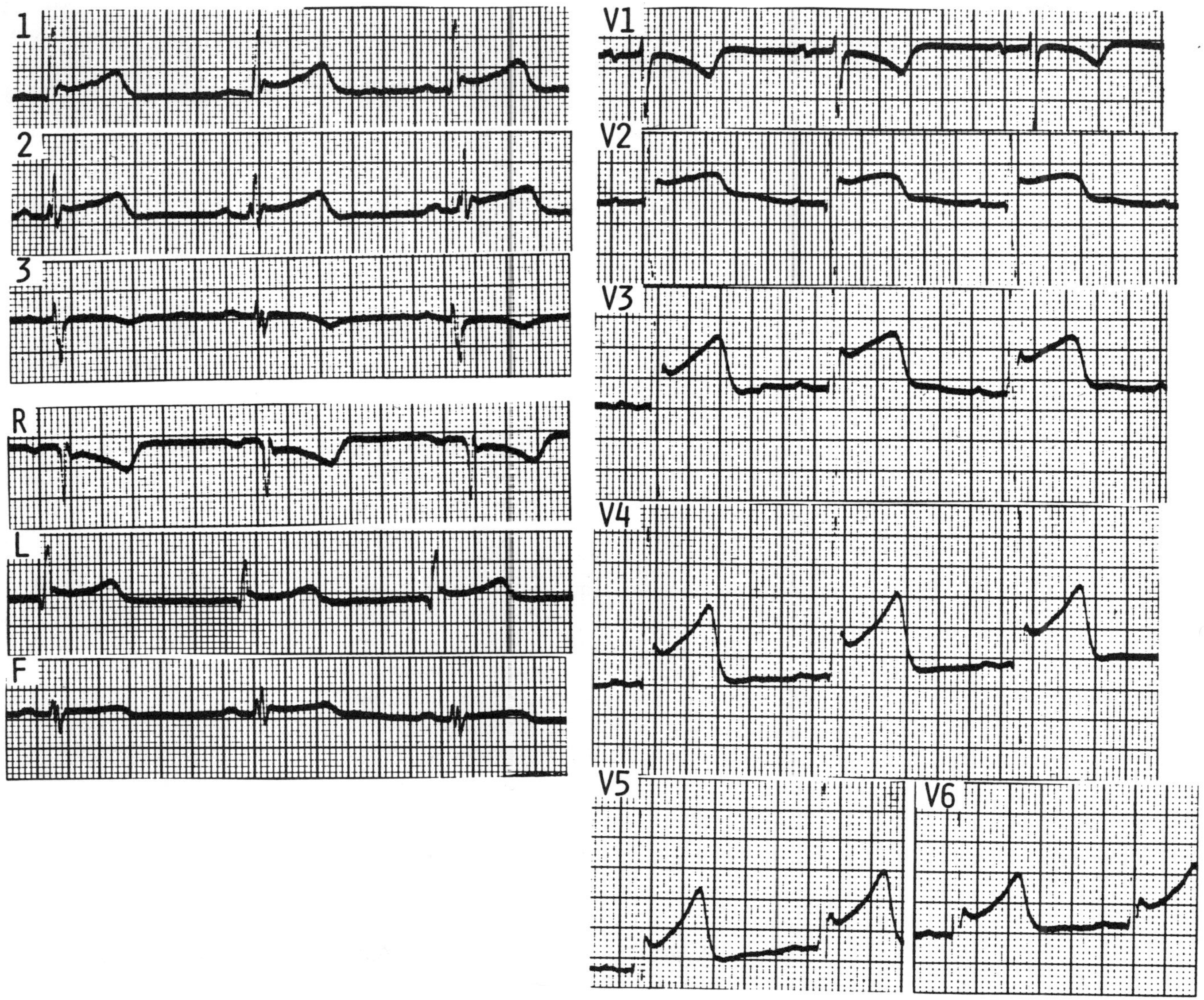


**Figure 28** The tracing is of a 33-year-old man. It was taken six days following craniotomy and frontal lobotomy.

# NUMBER 28 *Keep It Cool* Jorge I. Martinez-Lopez

## ELUCIDATION

The tracing shows typical findings seen in hypothermia. There is pronounced sinus bradycardia and QT interval prolongation. The terminal portion of the QRS complex is deformed by the characteristic "Osborn wave."

## DISCUSSION

The patient had a stormy postoperative course marked by coma and persistent hyperpyrexia. Because of the latter, an ice mattress was used intermittently to lower his rectal temperature to between 94°F and 98°F.

Total body hypothermia—accidental, spontaneous, or induced—is associated with a constellation of electrocardiographic alterations. Failure to recognize these abnormalities leads to erroneous interpretation of the electrocardiogram and to improper management. The electrocardiographic abnormalities are *reversible* with rewarming, with no apparent sequelae.

At core temperatures below 90°F, the firing rate of the SA node progressively slows down. This is followed by a gradual change in polarity of the T waves, and by prolongation of the P-R, QRS, and Q-T intervals.

Supraventricular and ventricular arrhythmias occur often. Atrial fibrillation and premature ventricular beats are frequent forerunners of ventricular fibrillation.

With more profound degrees of hypothermia, ventricular fibrillation may appear without warning or premonitory arrhythmias. In others, profound hypothermia may so depress atrioventricular and intraventricular conduction that cardiac activity ceases entirely.

The "Osborn wave"—also referred to as "J wave," "camel hump wave," and "hypothermic hump"—is the most distinctive landmark on the electrocardiogram with extreme degrees of hypothermia. The deflection is inscribed in the terminal portion of the QRS complex, deforming it, and is oriented in the same direction as the major deflection of the ventricular complex. The origin and clinical significance of the "Osborn wave" have not been clarified.

Recognition of the electrocardiographic abnormalities produced by total body hypothermia has important clinical implications. Patients showing these alterations are in imminent danger. Accordingly, measures designed to rewarm the patient should be promptly instituted.

## SELECTED READINGS

Clements SD Jr, Hurst JW: Diagnostic value of electrocardiographic abnormalities observed in subjects accidentally exposed to cold. *Am J Cardiol* 29:729, 1972.

Trevino A, Razi B, Beller M: The characteristic electrocardiogram of accidental hypothermia. *Arch Intern Med* 127:470, 1971.

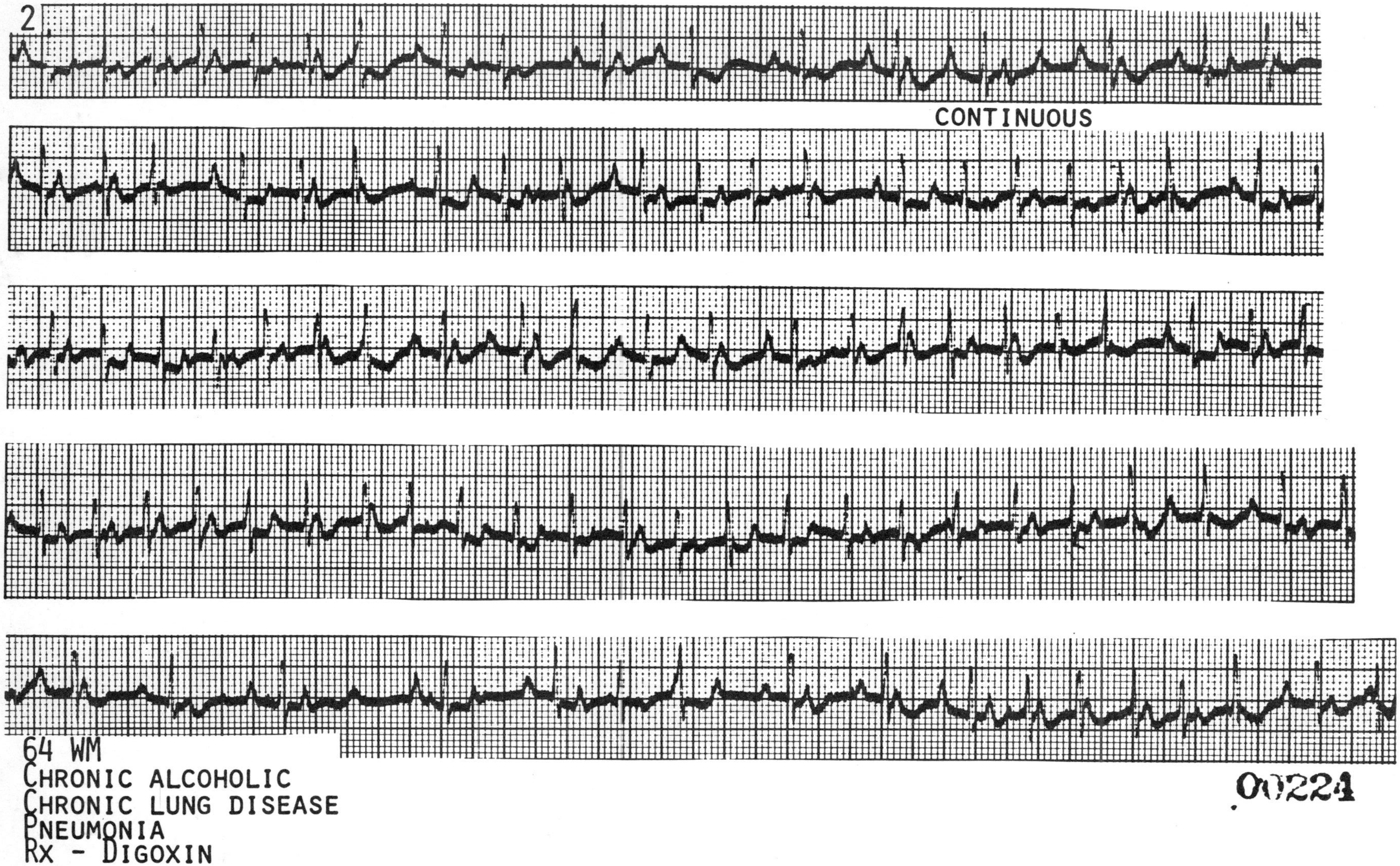


**Figure 29** The tracing is a continuous rhythm strip (lead II). It was taken on a 64-year-old man with the diagnoses of chronic alcoholism and chronic lung disease. He was taking digitalis.

# NUMBER 29 *Chaos in the Heart* Jorge I. Martinez-Lopez

## ELUCIDATION

**Diagnosis**—*Chaotic atrial tachycardia (CAT)*

The rhythm strip shows several features. Upright P waves of varied morphology (multifocal) are noted throughout. The P-P intervals and the P-R intervals are not constant. The atrial rate is rapid and also variable. Inverted P waves (fourth strip from the top) suggest atrial echo beats.

Ventricular complexes are narrow, indicating normal conduction of supraventricular impulses into the ventricular musculature. The ventricular response is grossly irregular.

## DISCUSSION

CAT, a distinctive electrocardiographic and clinical entity, probably occurs more often than generally realized. The principal electrocardiographic features are: 1) a rapid atrial rate, greater than 100 per minute; 2) changing P wave morphology, usually from at least three separate foci; 3) irregular P-P intervals; 4) variable P-R intervals; and 5) an isoelectric baseline between consecutive P waves. The variable P wave morphology or the "absence" of P waves when the mean atrial vector is perpendicular to the recording lead, combined with the irregular ventricular response, may lead to an erroneous interpretation of atrial fibrillation or atrial flutter "with variable A-V block." Other conditions that must be differentiated from CAT include sinus rhythm with multifocal atrial premature beats, wandering atrial pacemaker, and paroxysmal atrial tachycardia with block. Additional electrocardiographic alterations may be introduced by the underlying disorder and/or its management.

The infrequency with which the arrhythmia has been reported is likely related to its transient nature, so that it may escape detection, and to erroneous electrocardiographic interpretation. The commonest sequence is for the patient to have preexisting unifocal or multifocal atrial premature beats, then CAT, followed by progression to atrial fibrillation, or for atrial fibrillation to precede and follow the onset of CAT. In some patients, however, CAT develops without a preexisting disturbance of rhythm. Recurrences are common in all patients who exhibit CAT.

In ordinary "unifocal" paroxysmal atrial tachycardia, the evidence favors a re-entry pathway passing through the AV junction as the mechanism responsible for the arrhythmia. That is not the case in CAT, where the mechanism remains controversial. Some believe it to be similar to that of unifocal atrial tachycardia, except that more than one atrial ectopic focus is present (multifocal atrial tachycardia). Others have suggested that it is a re-entry type tachycardia, adding that "the re-entry circuit varies in duration as well as in its precise anatomic course from beat to beat because of areas of impaired conduction in the atria."

In what clinical setting is CAT seen? Almost all patients with the arrhythmia are elderly and, with few exceptions, severely ill with acute or chronic disorders, such as cor pulmonale, ischemic heart disease, cardiac failure, diabetes mellitus, or some combination of these factors. Although CAT has been reported in association with hypokalemia and following the use of aminophylline in patients with pulmonary disease, no causal relationship has been shown between the arrhythmia and digitalis toxicity. More rarely, a "benign" variety has been observed in healthy young individuals with otherwise normal hearts.

In the past, the prognosis for CAT has been considered serious. The reported mortality in patients with the arrhythmia is 50% to 60%. However, the rhythm disturbance itself is probably "benign." Although it occurred frequently in the seriously ill, death was *not* attributed to CAT but rather to the underlying disorder or its complications.

The need for treatment of CAT is dictated by the presence or absence of hemodynamic alterations. Because of its transiency and spontaneous conversion to other disturbances of rhythm, it does not often require therapy. In the unusual situation, when the duration of the arrhythmia is sufficiently prolonged or associated with rapid ventricular rate, treatment is needed.

Fundamental to control of CAT is improvement in the general clinical condition of the patient, including improved oxygenation, correction of metabolic abnormalities, and control of sepsis. The arrhythmia has been unresponsive to digitalis, quinidine, lidocaine, and diphenylhydantoin. Cardioversion may abolish it. The adage "Do not treat the ECG, treat *the patient* with the ECG abnormality" is certainly most applicable in this situation.

## SELECTED READINGS

D'Cruz IA, Mehta AB, et al: Benign repetitive multifocal atrial tachycardia: response to intracardiac atrial stimulation. *Am Heart J* 88:671–672, 1974.

Lipson MJ, Naimi S: Multifocal atrial tachycardia (chaotic atrial tachycardia): clinical associations and significance. *Circulation* 42:397–407, 1970.

Shine KI, Kastor JA, Yurchak PM: Multifocal atrial tachycardia: clinical and electrocardiographic features in 32 patients. *N Engl J Med* 279:344–349, 1968.

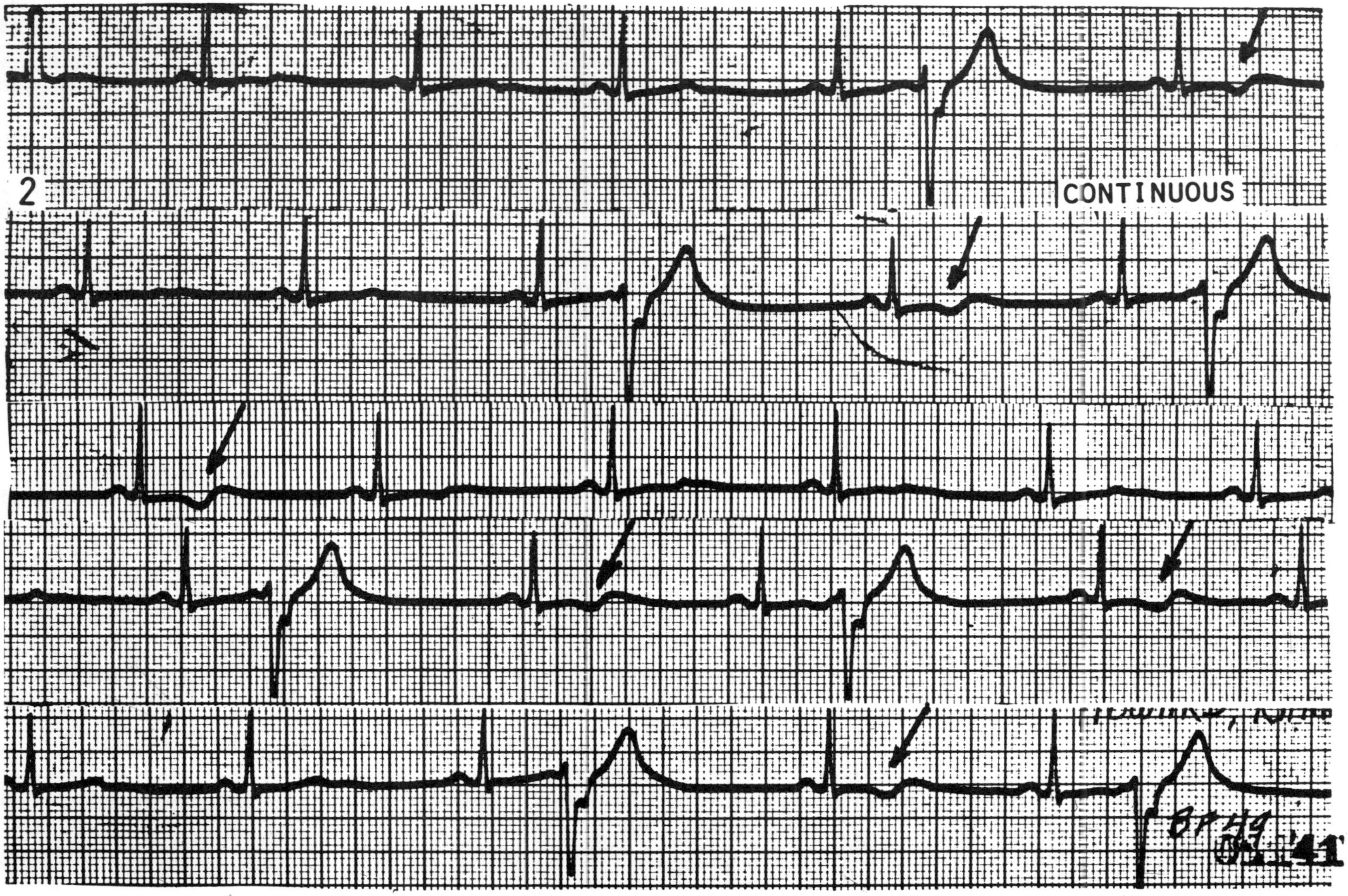


**Figure 30** The continuous tracing is of a 57-year-old man with systemic arterial hypertension. He was taking reserpine, hydrochlorothiazide, quinidine sulfate, and allopurinol orally.

# NUMBER 30 *Poor Man's Stress Test?* Jorge I. Martinez-Lopez

## ELUCIDATION

**Diagnosis—***Postextrasystolic T wave changes*

Sinus rhythm is present at a rate of 79 per minute. The P-R, QRS, and QT intervals are within normal limits. T waves are generally low, and prominent U waves are present.

The abnormal QRS complexes seen frequently represent ventricular premature beats associated with full compensatory pauses.

The prominent feature in the tracing is pointed out by the arrows: following every ventricular premature beat, the T wave of the first conducted beat after the pause is inverted. These are so-called *postextrasystolic T wave changes.*

## DISCUSSION

Of all the components of the ECG, the T wave, which represents ventricular repolarization, is the most labile. Ventricular repolarization is a process sensitive to a large number of physiological, pathological, and pharmacological influences. Therefore, the polarity, shape, and amplitude of the T wave can be affected by a wide variety of factors. For example, slight fluctuations from day to day in the size of the T wave in an individual are normal; hyperventilation and normal activities such as exercise, sleep, smoking, and the ingestion of a large meal may all result in some T wave changes. Pathologic conditions which can cause T wave abnormalities include all forms of cardiac disease, anemia, severe infections, acidosis, fever, anoxia, cerebral disorders, and many others. Among the pharmacologic agents which may alter the T wave are digitalis, potassium, emetine, and radiopaque material injected in the coronary arteries.

In spite of the recognized lability of the T wave, many attempts have been made to differentiate "benign" from "malignant" T wave changes with questionable degrees of success. At present, there is no specific way to establish this distinction; T wave changes *alone* must be regarded as a nonspecific finding. This advice must be heeded especially when carrying out graded exercise "stress" tests; development of abnormal T waves during and/or after graded exercise stress *does not* constitute an abnormal response when not accompanied by any other changes in the ECG.

T-wave changes occurring in the first conducted beat following a ventricular premature beat (VPB), however, have been the subject of considerable speculation since first described in 1915. Commonly designated as the postextrasystolic T-wave change (PE-T), it has also been frivolously referred to as the "poor man's stress test." This last term implies that it has an ominous significance. But does it? Does this uncommon phenomenon uncover "silent" heart disease, specifically coronary artery disease, as has been suggested?

Recent studies, summarized below, have provided valuable data regarding PE-T, but have failed to disclose its mechanism. Studies in which premature beats were mechanically induced showed that the most premature contraction was followed by the most prominent postextrasystolic contraction, which in turn was associated with the most prominent PE-T on the electrogram or surface ECG. Clearly, the "coupling ratio" plays a prominent role on PE-T. In addition, clinical recognition of PE-T relates at least in part to the amplitude of the preceding T wave itself. Hence it is obvious that PE-T is to be anticipated under *normal* circumstances in individuals with normal hearts, and not only following VPBs, but supraventricular premature beats as well.

Is PE-T observed more frequently in patients with heart disease? The evidence seems to indicate that it is. Experimental studies in which myocardial depressants were used demonstrated a relatively greater postextrasystolic contractile change and a relatively more marked PE-T; positive inotropic agents had a reverse effect. Hence, the contractile state of the myocardium also appears to play a role in determining the presence or absence of PE-T.

Finally, can PE-T be used to evaluate coronary artery disease and cardiac status? The significance of PE-T was assessed by coronary and left ventricular angiography by Engel et al. In their study, patients with normal coronary arteries were just as likely to have PE-T as patients with angiographically-shown CAD; changes were most frequently seen in the precordial leads. There was no correlation between PE-T and presence or absence of regional left ventricular asynergy, the left ventricular end-diastolic pressure, or the ejection fraction. They concluded that PE-T "cannot be used to diagnose or to localize coronary artery disease."

Poor man's stress test? Not so.

## SELECTED READINGS

Edmands RE, Bailey JC: The postextrasystolic T wave change. *Am J Cardiol* 28:536, 1971.

Engel TR, et al: Postextrasystolic T wave changes and angiographic coronary disease. *Br Heart J* 39:371, 1977.

Levine HD, et al: The clinical significance of postextrasystolic T wave changes. *Circulation* 6:538, 1952.

Mann RH, Burchell RB: The significance of T wave inversion following ventricular extrasystoles. *Am Heart J* 47:504, 1954.

White PD: Alternation of the pulse: a common clinical condition. *Am J Med Sci* 150:82, 1915.

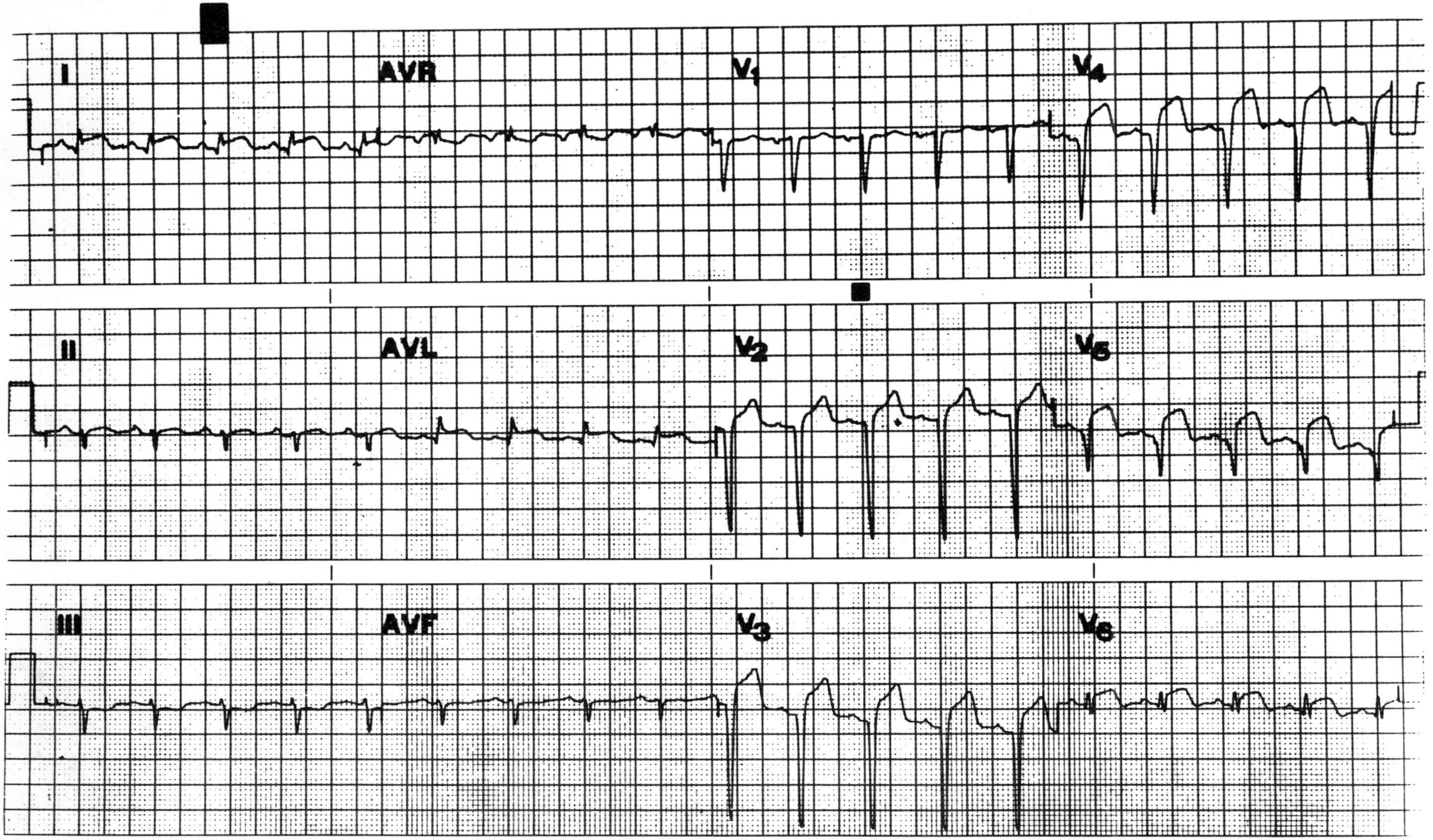


**Figure 31** This ECG was recorded from a 48-year-old man six months after an acute myocardial infarction. He was limited with angina, dyspnea, and fatigue at the time the ECG was obtained.

## NUMBER 31 *Battle of the Bulge* Stephen P. Glasser

### ELUCIDATION

The ECG demonstrates a large anterolateral myocardial infarction with persistent ST segment elevation and T wave inversion. Left anterior hemiblock and left atrial enlargement are also present. X-ray and left ventricular angiography demonstrated a large anterolateral left ventricular aneurysm. On coronary angiography, the left anterior descending coronary artery was completely occluded just distal to the first septal perforator. One week prior to planned surgery the patient was admitted in cardiogenic shock and died.

### DISCUSSION

Recently, the definition of left ventricular aneurysm has been modified from the classic description of an outpouching of endo-, myo-, and epicardium (now called dyskinesis) to any area of noncontractile myocardium (akinesis) or poorly contractile myocardium (asynchrony and asyneresis). Of interest is that the classic diskinetic aneurysm generally takes a mean of three years to develop, whereas in our patient, dyskinesis was in evidence within eight weeks following the infarction. The classic symptoms related to left ventricular aneurysm are those of congestive heart failure, angina pectoris, ventricular arrhythmia, and embolic phenomena. When refractory to medical treatment, these are also the indications for surgical excision. These symptoms can be related to the aneurysm via several pathophysiologic mechanisms. With systole, blood fills the expanding aneurysm, thereby decreasing forward ejection much the same way that mitral regurgitation does. Additionally, the remaining normal myocardium must increase its fiber length in order to maintain stroke volume, but this occurs at the expense of an increase in myocardial $O_2$ demand. Also, compliance in the wall of the aneurysm is usually decreased so that left ventricular filling is also reduced.

Electrocardiographically, ventricular aneursym is important from two aspects: its diagnostic changes and its association with intractable arrhythmia. Diagnostically, it has been stated that R-ST segment elevation persisting more than six months after myocardial infarction is suggestive of ventricular aneurysm. Recently, Mills et al concluded that ST-segment elevation after myocardial infarction resolved within two weeks in 95% of inferior but only 40% of anterior infarctions, and that if ST-segment elevation persisted more than two weeks it tended not to resolve subsequently. Miller et al found that in patients with ECG evidence of transmural infarction, concomitant ST elevation with T wave inversion was indicative of asynergy in 95% of patients, while dyskinesis was present in 68% of patients. Bodenheimer et al demonstrated left ventricular aneurysms in 22% of patients without pathologic Q waves. Overall, it can probably be said that in patients with coronary artery disease, persistent ST-segment elevation two weeks or more after myocardial infarction is a specific but not an ultrasensitive index of asynergy.

From the aspect of its association with arrhythmias, there have now been a number of reports of medically intractable rhythm disturbances cured by aneurysmectomy, but surprisingly little is known about the mechanism. Gallagher et al utilized epicardial mapping techniques to demonstrate that the site of origin of the ventricular arrhythmia was at the margin of the ventricular aneurysm, although they were unable to determine whether the site was located in the endocardium or intramurally.

### SELECTED READINGS


Arkin BM, Hueter DC, Ryan TJ: Predictive value of electrocardiographic patterns in localizing left ventricular asynergy in coronary artery disease. *Am Heart J* 97:453, 1979.

Helfant RH, Bodenheimer MM, Banka VS: Q waves, myocardial fibrosis, and asynergy. *Cardiovasc Med* September 1979, p 1001.

Keikkila J, Neiminen M: Echoventriculographic detection, localization, and quantification of left ventricular asynergy in acute myocardial infarction. *Br Heart J* 37:46, 1975.

Miller RR, Amsterdam EA, Bogren HG, et al: Electrocardiographic and cineangiographic correlations in assessment of the location, nature and extent of abnormal left ventricular segmental contraction in coronary artery disease. *Circulation* 49:447, 1974.

Raskoff W, Smith, GL, Jr, Dymnicka SK, et al: Sensitivity and specificity of electrocardiographic diagnosis of ventricular motion disorders. *Chest* 69:148, 1976.

# NUMBER 32 *Up, Up, and Away* Pamela I. Clark, Stephen P. Glasser

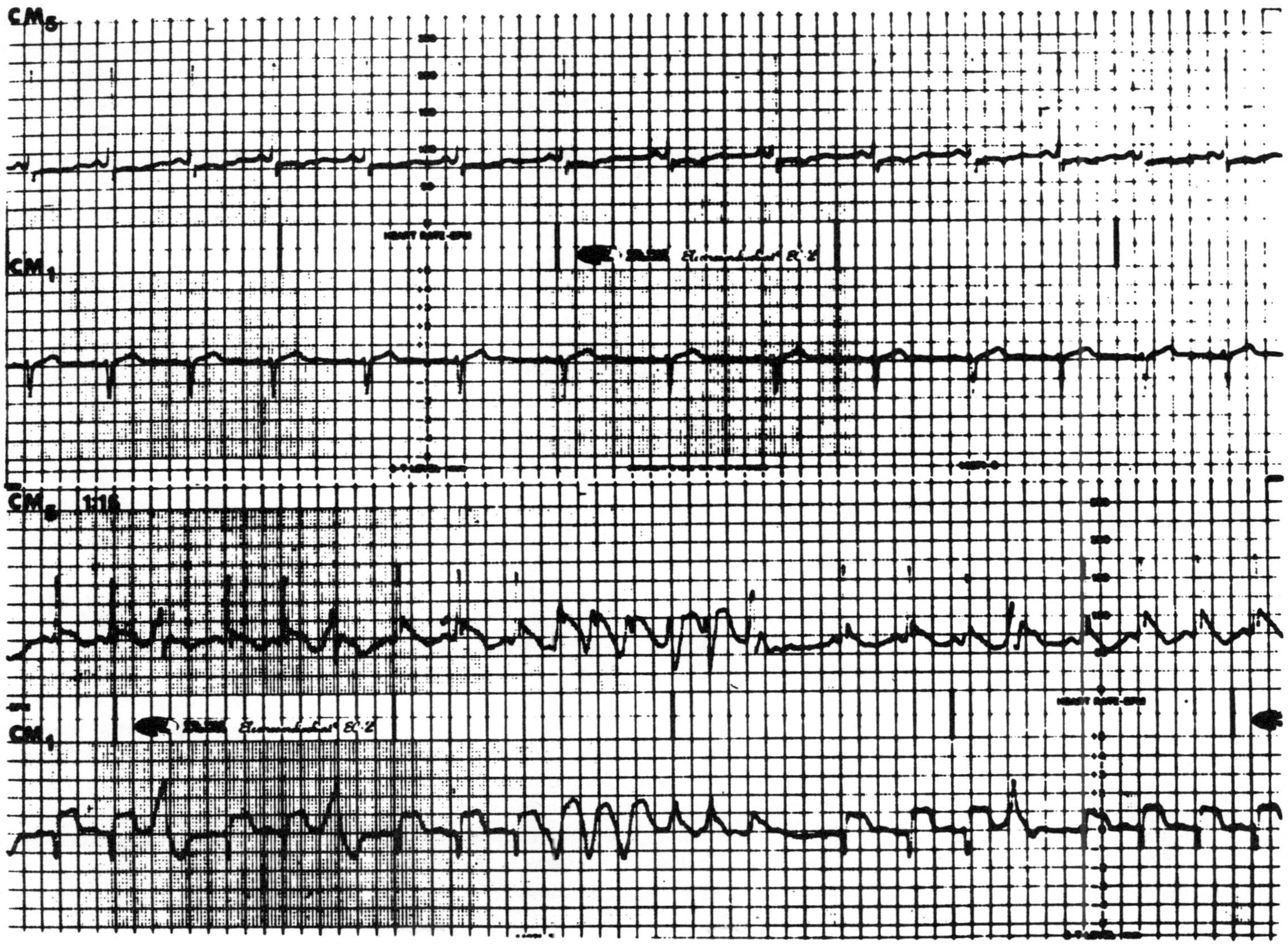


**Figure 32** A 54-year-old salesman was evaluated for oppressive substernal chest pain which occurred 5 to 6 times daily, primarily at rest, and rarely with exertion. The rhythm strips are from an ambulatory (Holter) recording.

# NUMBER 32 *Up, Up, and Away* Pamela I. Clark, Stephen P. Glasser

## ELUCIDATION

**Diagnosis**—*Prinzmetal's variant angina*

The baseline tracings show 1-mm S-T segment elevation in the modified $V_1$ lead and 1-mm horizontal depression in the modified $V_5$ lead. At 1:15 AM the subject awakened with chest pain. At that time, he showed 6-mm S-T elevation in $V_1$ and 3-mm S-T elevation in $V_5$, as well as multiform ventricular ectopic beats and a burst of ventricular tachycardia.

## DISCUSSION

Classic angina pectoris is typically induced by exertion and relieved by rest. When spontaneous angina occurs at rest, exercise capacity is usually already greatly limited, and severe multivessel obstructive coronary disease is usually present. In 1959 Prinzmetal described a variant anginal syndrome in which attacks of pain recurred almost exclusively at rest, were rarely provoked by exercise, and were associated with transient S-T segment elevation (in contrast to the S-T segment depression usually seen during episodes of classic angina). The diagnosis of Prinzmetal's variant angina can be suspected, therefore, by the history, and confirmed by the demonstration of S-T segment elevation during an attack. While such confirmation can sometimes be obtained by recording an ECG promptly during an anginal episode, ambulatory (Holter) monitoring provides a unique opportunity to detect transient S-T segment elevation. The use of ambulatory monitoring with the accompanying diary of activities and symptoms has shown, too, that S-T elevation often occurs in individuals with Prinzmetal's angina at times when they are having no anginal symptoms.

Not all episodes of S-T segment elevation seen during ambulatory monitoring are associated with Prinzmetal's angina. S-T segment elevation has been documented in individuals with apparent neurocirculatory asthenia, following myocardial infarction, with ventricular aneurysm, and in unstable or preinfarction angina. The clinical history should help to differentiate these conditions.

Certain conditions should be fulfilled before relying on ambulatory monitoring techniques to reliably detect S-T segment shifts. The low frequency response of the recording system must be adequate to faithfully record the S-T segment. A relatively stable baseline must be present. And the QRS complexes during S-T segment shifts should closely resemble in magnitude and direction those complexes preceding the event (this helps to minimize confusion resulting from postural changes and ectopic rhythms). Additionally, the ability to record at least two precordial leads greatly enhances the reliability of data obtained.

## SELECTED READINGS

Golding B, et al: Transient S-T elevations detected by 24-hour ECG monitoring during normal daily activity. *Am Heart J* 86:501–507, 1973.

Guazzi M, Fiorentini C, Polese A, et al: Continuous electrocardiographic recording in Prinzmetal's variant angina pectoris. *Br Heart J* 32:611–616, 1970.

Prinzmetal M, Kennamer R, Merliss R, et al: Angina pectoris. I. A variant form of angina pectoris: preliminary report. *Am J Med* 27:375, 1959.

## NUMBER 33 *Uncommon Cause for Pause* Stephen P. Glasser, Pamela I. Clark

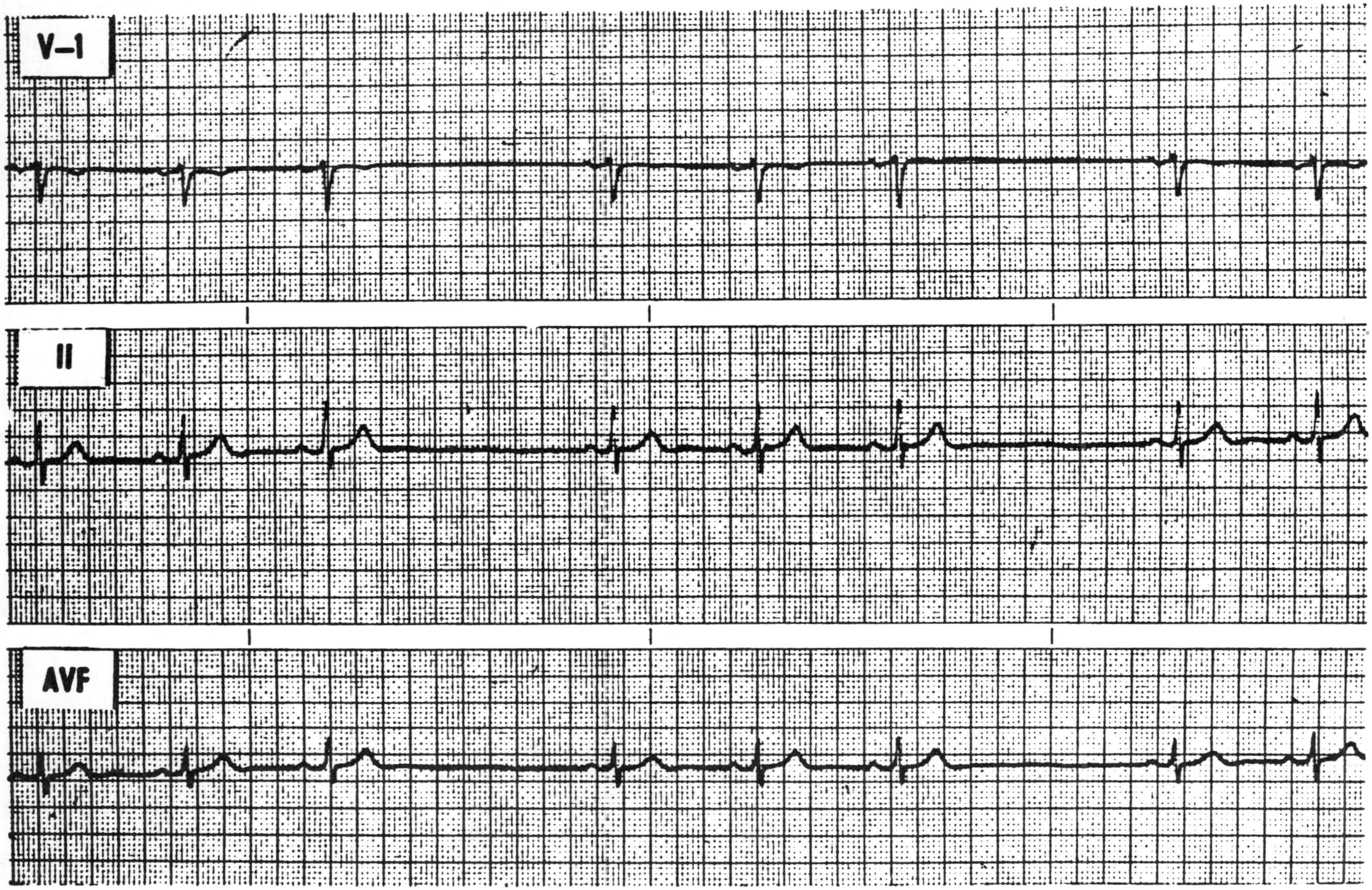


**Figure 33** The rhythm strip was recorded from a 59-year-old man who complained of dizziness.

## NUMBER 33 *Uncommon Cause for Pause* Stephen P. Glasser, Pamela I. Clark

### ELUCIDATION

The rhythm strip (simultaneous leads $V_1$, II, and AVF) shows a relatively uncommon cause of a pause: sinoatrial block. The first three beats are normal sinus beats, followed by failure of the next sinus cycle to be manifest. The resulting pause is exactly twice the preceding cycle length.

### DISCUSSION

Formation of the normal sinus impulse is not demonstrated by standard ECG. Only when the impulse is transmitted to the atria is the electrocardiographic P wave inscribed. The rhythm strip shows sinus rhythm with sudden failure of a P wave (and ensuing QRS-T waves) to appear at the time expected. The sinus node is presumed to have fired on schedule, but the impulse is blocked at the sinoatrial junction, never reaching the surrounding atrial myocardium.

Sinoatrial (SA) block may be manifested as first-, second-, or third-degree block, as are the more familiar AV blocks. First-degree block or delayed exit of the impulse from the sinus node to the surrounding tissue is virtually impossible to detect on standard ECG. Third-degree or complete sinus node exit block, in which no P waves are written, cannot be distinguished from sinus arrest, that is, from total failure of sinus impulse formation. But the second-degree blocks, Mobitz type I (Wenckebach) and Mobitz type II, leave characteristic electrocardiographic footprints. Sinoatrial block of the Wenckebach type results in progressively shorter P-P intervals until a P wave is dropped. The resulting pause is not a multiple of the preceding P-P interval. This is analogous to A-V nodal Wenckebach in which the R-R intervals shorten until a QRS is dropped, and the resulting pause is not a multiple of the preceding R-R interval. Sinoatrial block of the Mobitz II type is diagnosed by constant P-P intervals followed by a pause that is exactly twice the preceding cycle length.

Sinoatrial block is seen in organic cardiac disease, but may be a manifestation of digitalis or quinidine toxicity. If drug withdrawal fails to resolve the dysrhythmia, atropine or isoproterenol may fascilitate sinoatrial conduction. Permanent cardiac pacing may be necessary for the patient with persistent symptoms.

### SELECTED READINGS

Myerburg RJ: Electrocardiographic diagnosis of sinus node rhythm variations and S-A block, in Schlant RC, Hurst JW (eds): *Advances in Electrocardiography.* New York, Grune & Stratton Inc, 1972, pp 77–80.

Shamroth L: *The Disorders of Cardiac Rhythm.* Oxford, Blackwell Scientific Publications Ltd, 1971, pp 193–195.

## NUMBER 34 *Seven-Year "Switch"* Stephen P. Glasser, Pamela I. Clark

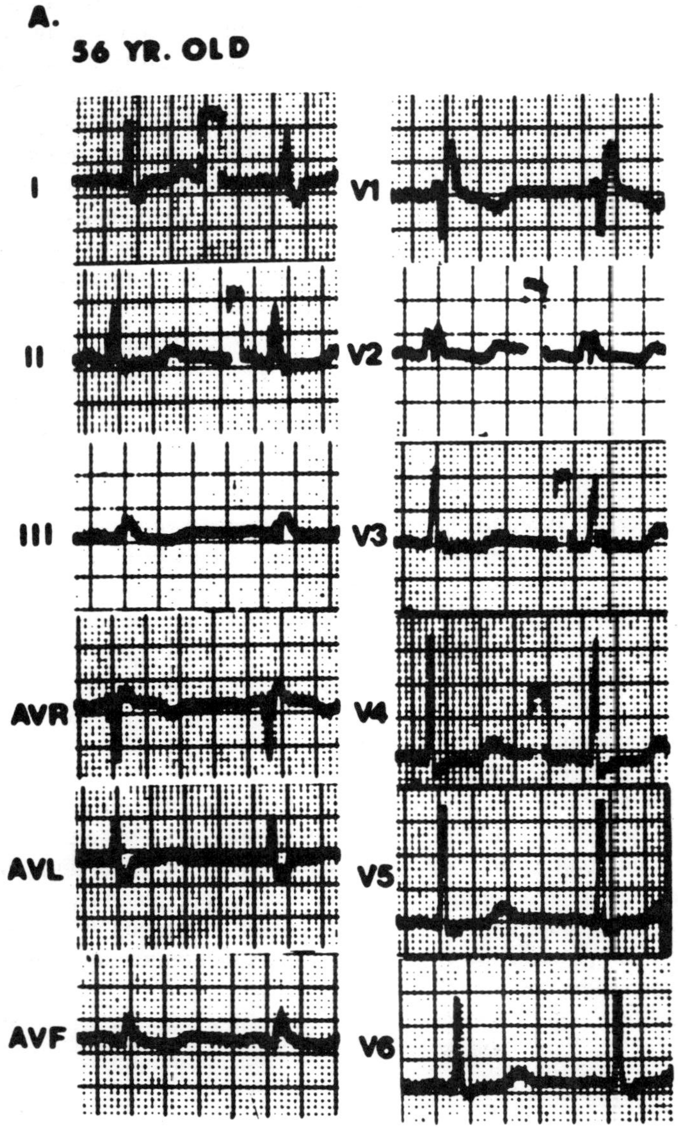


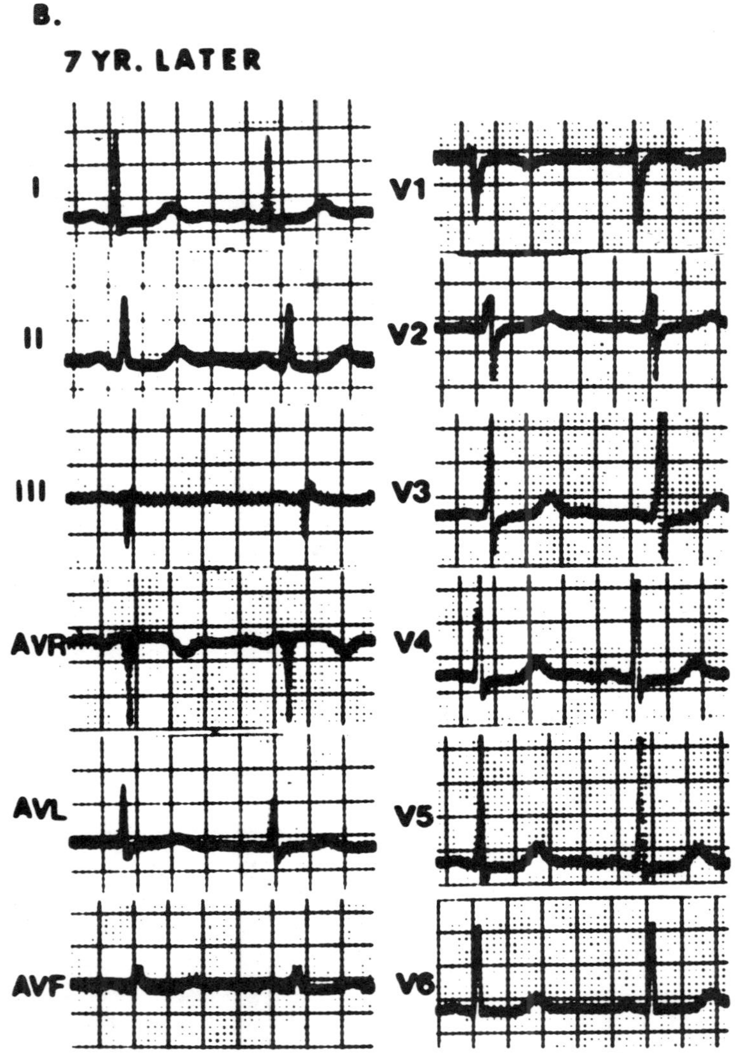


**Figure 34-1** Recorded from a 56-year-old woman without cardiovascular symptoms. **Figure 34-2** Recorded from the same patient seven years later.

# NUMBER 34 *Seven-Year "Switch"* Stephen P. Glasser, Pamela I. Clark

## ELUCIDATION

This is a case of right bundle branch block (RBBB) which persisted for seven years, then spontaneously returned to normal conduction. The panel on the left shows the classic criteria for RBBB: normal initial QRS forces, but abnormal late QRS forces (wide S wave in I, AVL, and $V_6$, and tall R′ in $V_1$), producing a QRS width of 0.14 second. The panel on the right shows normal QRS width of 0.08 second and the return of normal QRS terminal forces. One explanation for the resolution of the conduction abnormality would be that it had been heart rate related. A rapid rate was achieved with amyl nitrite inhalation, and sinus slowing was achieved by carotid sinus massage and Valsalva's maneuver, but the normal conduction pattern persisted.

## DISCUSSION

Transient and intermittent bundle branch blocks are well recognized. It is, however, generally accepted that once constant bundle branch block has been established, it remains permanent.

Bauer emphasized that bundle branch block can no longer be regarded as a stable condition always associated with an organic lesion interrupting the main bundle branches. Cases have been reported in which normal conduction could be induced by a variety of maneuvers including deep inspiration, carotid sinus stimulation, and pharmacologic agents. Generally, more rapid rates induce abnormal conduction; but occasional cases of brady-dependent bundle branch blocks have been described.

Kalett reported a case of left bundle branch block with remission after four years. The present case is of interest because it is one of the longest cases of a constant bundle branch block that we are aware of with spontaneous disappearance. It is shown to be unrelated to rate altering or vagal maneuvers.

## SELECTED READINGS


Bauer GE: Transient bundle branch block. *Circulation* 29:730, 1964.

Kalett J: Bundle branch block with spontaneous remission after four years. *Am Heart J* 29:120, 1945.

Massumi RA: Bradycardia-dependent bundle branch block. *Circulation* 38:1066, 1968.

Scott RC: Clinical assessment of left bundle branch block. *Am Heart J* 70:535, 1965.

# NUMBER 35 *Pseudoinfarction* Stephen P. Glasser, Pamela I. Clark

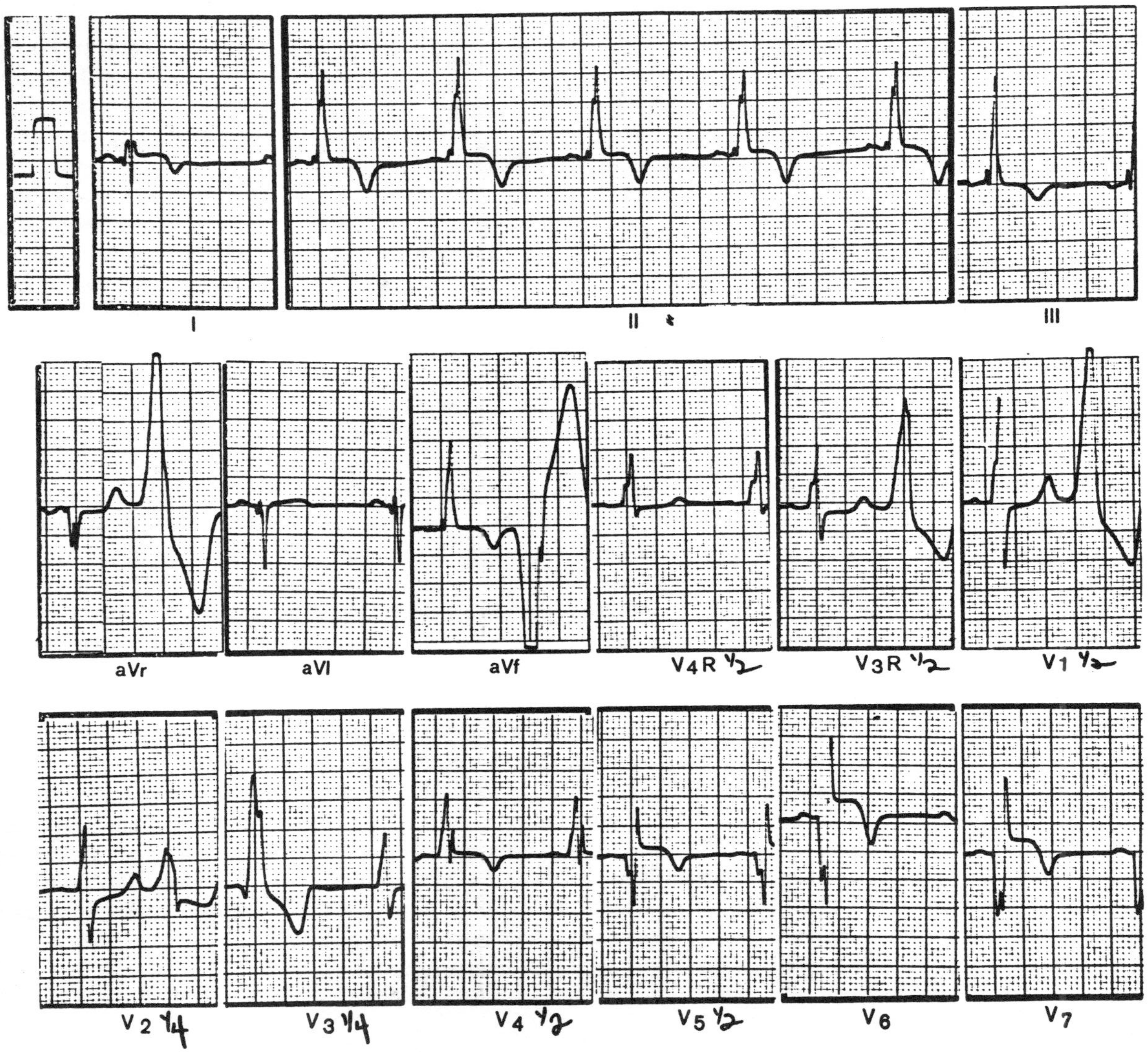


**Figure 35** The patient was a 12-year-old girl noted to have a murmur at age 3. She has had several episodes of congestive heart failure and intermittent chest pain.

## NUMBER 35 *Pseudoinfarction* Stephen P. Glasser, Pamela I. Clark

### ELUCIDATION

The ECG demonstrates ventricular premature beats, left ventricular hypertrophy, intraventricular conduction defect, and the pattern of anterolateral infarction. In this case it represents a pseudoinfarction pattern.

### DISCUSSION

Most of the ECG abnormalities reported in patients with idiopathic hypertrophic stenosis (IHSS) are those which could be anticipated in the presence of left ventricular outflow obstruction, namely, left ventricular hypertrophy and left atrial enlargement. Left ventricular hypertrophy and left atrial enlargement are seen in about 75% of patients with IHSS. Other reported abnormalities are the Wolff-Parkinson-White syndrome (WPW) and abnormally deep and broad septal Q waves.

Braunwald et al reported deep Q waves in 16 of 64 patients (25%) with IHSS. In the past, there was no definite evidence to indicate whether these Q waves were due to attendant coronary artery disease and infarction, although a number of these occurred in age groups in which coronary disease was unlikely. Subsequently, there has been further validation with coronary arteriography that Q waves present in IHSS frequently occur without concomitant coronary disease. Two patterns of pseudoinfarction have been demonstrated: a pattern of inferior myocardial infarction and a pattern of anterolateral infarction. In both instances, it has been suggested that the pseudoinfarction pattern is a result of electromotive forces generated from the asymmetric septal hypertrophy unbalanced by the forces generated from the free left ventricular wall. Although it is suggested that this pattern (as well as the WPW pattern) is more common in the familial rather than the nonfamilial form of IHSS, no other explanation is apparent as to why some patients manifest this ECG pattern while others do not.

Other ECG abnormalities reported in IHSS, but which are not specific or characteristic, include left axis deviation (20%), ST-T wave abnormalities (90% to 100%), and right ventricular hypertrophy (presumably the result of subpulmonic right ventricular outflow obstruction). Interestingly, conduction defects and atrial arrhythmias are not common. Left bundle branch block, a pattern one might think should be common, occurred in only 1 of 64 patients in the study by Braunwald et al.

### SELECTED READINGS


Braunwald E, Lambrew CT, Rockoff SD, et al: Idiopathic hypertrophic subaortic stenosis. *Circulation* 29–30(suppl 4):20–29, 1974.

Wigle ED, Baron RH: The electrocardiogram in muscular subaortic stenosis—effect of a left septal incision and right bundle-branch block. *Circulation* 34:585–593, 1966.

## NUMBER 36 *The Breaking Point* Stephen P. Glasser, Pamela I. Clark

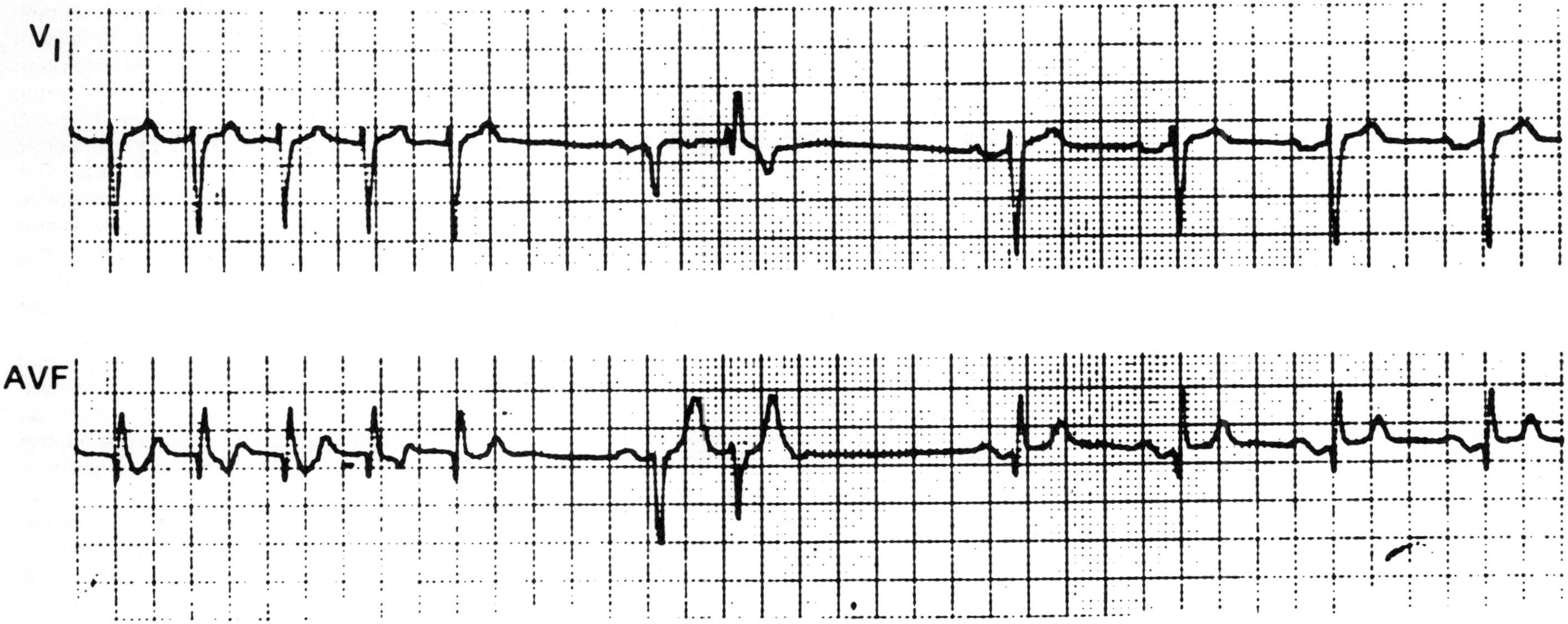


**Figure 36** A 52-year-old woman had a sudden onset of palpitations and weakness. She had no known prior cardiovascular problems and was taking no medications. Examination revealed a blood pressure of 95/70 mm Hg and a heart rate of 140. A question of a diastolic murmur was noted. The ECG was recorded during carotid sinus massage.

# NUMBER 36 *The Breaking Point* Stephen P. Glasser, Pamela I. Clark

## ELUCIDATION

A regular rhythm at a rate of 140 beats per minute is present with no obviously apparent P waves. The narrow QRS complex is compatible with a supraventricular rhythm. The impression of inferior wall ST segment abnormality is given. Midway through the tracing (during conversion) a pause of 1000 msec is followed by an apparent sinus beat, then an atrial premature beat (both beats are conducted aberrantly, the first with left anterior fascicular block and the second with incomplete right bundle branch block), and finally restoration of sinus rhythm. Note that the S-T segment changes present during the tachyarrhythmia disappear with the last beat of the tachyarrhythmia (5th beat), and that the S-T segment changes are not present in the immediate postconversion sinus rhythm. This documents the presence of atrial depolarization deforming the S-T segment of the first seven beats.

The tracing represents a supraventricular tachycardia (probably junctional) with conversion to sinus rhythm. A left atrial abnormality is present in the postconversion rhythm.

## DISCUSSION

A number of interesting phenomena are present in this tracing. The S-T segment abnormality suggesting myocardial ischemia is seen during the tachyarrhythmia and disappears with conversion to sinus rhythm. It has been suggested that the S-T segment depression frequently seen with sustained atrial tachyarrhythmias is the result of shortened diastolic filling time which abbreviates coronary blood flow, resulting in true myocardial ischemia. Another explanation is that the tachyarrhythmia somehow results in an abnormal repolarization sequence unrelated to ischemia. It is known, for instance, that the return of sinus rhythm following the termination of artificial pacing can be associated with repolarization abnormalities which persist for hours to months. Regardless of the mechanism, S-T segment abnormalities should be interpreted with caution when occurring during tachycardia or immediately after conversion to sinus rhythm, unless associated, with ischemic correlates (true angina, symptomatic hypotension, etc). Failure to do so may erroneously label a patient as having coronary artery disease. In the figure shown, an ''ischemic mechanism'' is not pertinent because the S-T segment deformity is caused by the presence of atrial depolarization, resulting in pseudo S-T changes.

Another interesting feature of this electrocardiogram is the appearance of aberrant beats in the immediate postconversion period. This is a form of the Ashman phenomenon, an abnormality of supraventricular conduction described in 1947. Ashman noted that aberrant ventricular conduction tends to occur in early (premature) beats (ie, those with short coupling intervals) following a long ventricular cycle (R-R interval). Although most frequently seen in atrial fibrillation because of its varying R-R and coupling intervals, the phenomenon can occur with any cardiac rhythm. Aberration must be differentiated from ventricular premature beats, and a number of criteria exist to help make this distinction. In the tracing shown, there should be little cause for confusion, however. The first postconversion beat is preceded by a P wave, and the second presumably has a prematurely occurring P wave which may be hidden in the T wave of the first beat. Although the usual form of aberration is that of a complete right bundle branch block (the right bundle has the longest refractory period), all forms of bundle branch and fascicular block patterns have been described.

Finally, the left atrial abnormality seen during the postconversion rhythm persisted, but caution is warranted in the interpretation of such abnormalities in this setting as they, too, may represent a temporary phenomenon.

In this case, the left atrial abnormality was significant, and was associated with a diastolic rumble of mitral stenosis which was easily auscultated in the presence of sinus rhythm. Thus, careful inspection of the conversion of tachyarrhythmias to sinus rhythm (the breaking point) can be extremely helpful in diagnosis and in the prevention of misdiagnosis.

## SELECTED READINGS

Chatterjee K, Harris A, Davies G, et al: Electrocardiographic changes subsequent to artificial ventricular depolarization. *Br Heart J* 31:770, 1969.

Gouaux JL, Ashman R: Auricular fibrillation with aberration simulating ventricular paroxysmal tachycardia. *Am Heart J* 34:366, 1947.

Marriott HJL, Sandler IA: Criteria, old and new, for differentiating between ectopic ventricular beats and aberrant ventricular conduction in the presence of atrial fibrillation. *Prog Cardiovasc Dis* 9:18, 1966.

## NUMBER 37 *Two-Way T Waves* Pamela I. Clark, Stephen P. Glasser

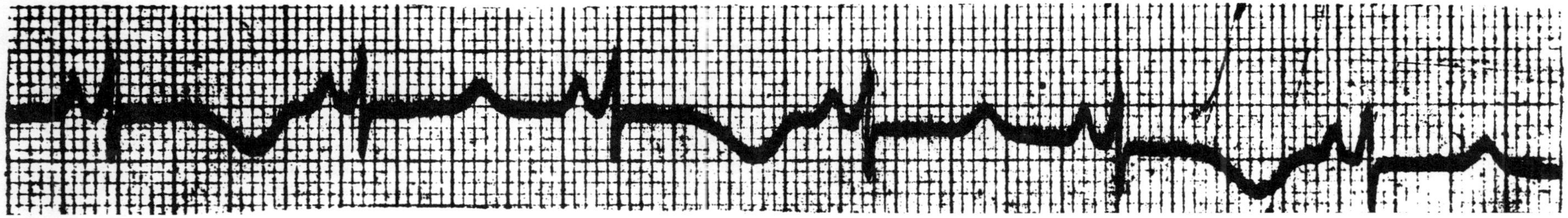

**Figure 37** This tracing was from a 70-year-old woman with the Guillain-Barré syndrome who had a respiratory arrest and required prolonged respiratory support. The tracing was recorded following resuscitation from an apparently spontaneous ventricular fibrillation. She had been countershocked to normal sinus rhythm without return of consciousness.

## NUMBER 37 *Two-Way T Waves* Pamela I. Clark, Stephen P. Glasser

### ELUCIDATION

The tracing shows sinus rhythm with regular R-R intervals, a constant pattern of depolarization, markedly prolonged Q-T intervals, and alternating size and polarity of every other T wave.

### DISCUSSION

Isolated T wave alternans is a rare and poorly understood phenomenon. The actual incidence is not known: 13 cases of acquired T wave alternans have been reported in the literature since its first description in 1913. Most reports have been in the form of isolated case studies. Those studies present a wide variety of clinical settings, and a definite common etiologic factor for all cases has not been identified. Possible contributing mechanisms that have been implicated include hypocalcemia, hypomagnesemia, hypokalemia, bradycardia, drug effect, and an autonomic nervous system mechanism. It is generally agreed that T wave alternans is a manifestation of alternans of the transmembrane action potential.

Common among most reported cases is the presence of severe heart disease. We have seen four cases of isolated T wave alternans, of which only one had evidence of primary cardiac disease.

The patient reported here was a usually active and well 70-year-old woman with a three-day history of progressive weakness, followed by ascending paralysis. Complete neurological work-up strongly suggested the Guillain-Barré syndrome. She experienced respiratory arrest, requiring prolonged respiratory support. She had an apparently spontaneous ventricular fibrillation which responded to countershock. Several hours following resumption of normal sinus rhythm without resumption of consciousness, she demonstrated the alternans described above. The phenomenon was transitory, lasting approximately 30 minutes, and was not seen to recur. Arterial blood gases at the time of alternans were optimal, and serum sodium, potassium, chloride, $CO_2$ capacity, calcium, and magnesium levels were within normal limits. She had been given procainamide and a single intravenous dose of digoxin, 0.5 mg.

The patient never regained consciousness. Serial EEGs showed progressive, diffuse brain damage and, despite supportive therapy, she died 52 days after admission.

This patient, as well as three others whom we saw in a year's time, were all admitted to medical services other than cardiology, and were seen serendipitously by us. T wave alternans may be a less rare phenomenon than previously thought. Continued recognition and reporting of the pattern when it occurs may help to elucidate its etiology and clinical significance.

### SELECTED READINGS

Kimura E, Yoshida K: A case showing electrical alternans of the T wave without change in the QRS complex. *Am Heart J* 64:391, 1963.

Navarro-Lopez F, Cinca J, Sanz G, et al: Isolated T wave alternans. *Am Heart J* 95:369, 1978.

Rickets HN, Denison EK, Haywood LJ: Unusual T wave abnormality. Repolarization alternans associated with hypomagnesemia, acute alcoholism and cardiomyopathy. *JAMA* 207:365, 1969.

Surawicz B: The pathogenesis and clinical significance of primary T wave abnormalities, in Schlant RC, Hurst JW (eds): *Advances in Electrocardiography*. New York, Grune & Stratton, 1972.

## NUMBER 38 *Heartbreak or Headache?* Stephen P. Glasser, Pamela I. Clark

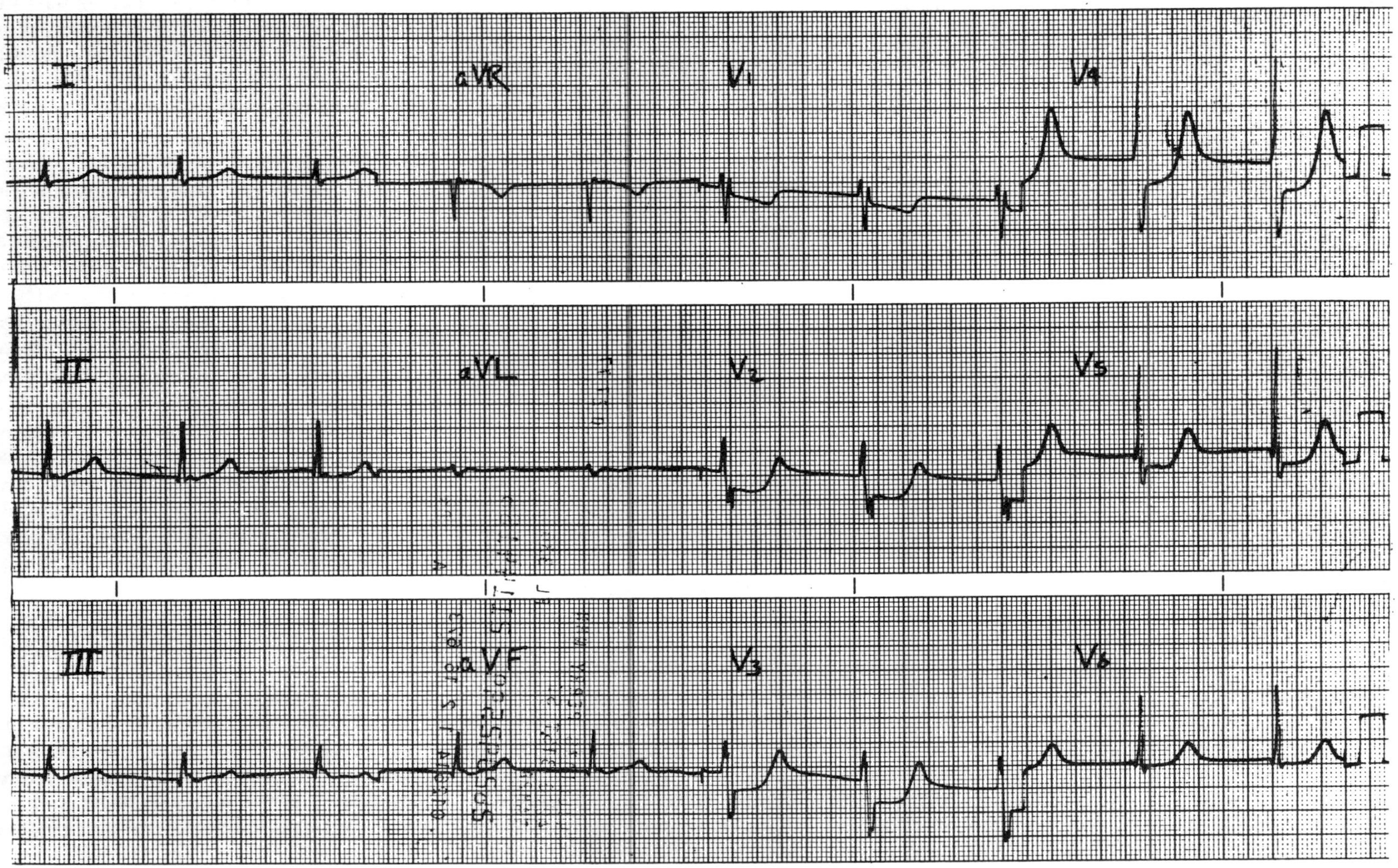


**Figure 38** The patient whose electrocardiogram is shown was a 56-year-old man admitted to the hospital with profound hypotension and semicoma secondary to overzealous antihypertensive therapy. Serum electrolytes were normal and the patient was not taking any additional medications. After several hours, blood pressure was restored and his ECG returned to its previous pattern of left ventricular hypertrophy and normal sinus rhythm.

## ELUCIDATION

The ECG demonstrates marked ST-T wave changes, prolonged Q-T interval of 560 msec, and an AV junctional rhythm. These abnormalities were thought to be secondary to his transient cerebral insufficiency, and resolved with normalization of his blood pressure.

## DISCUSSION

Striking abnormalities of ST-T waves have been known to occur in the presence of a variety of central nervous system diseases including stroke, trauma, tumor, and infection. The wave form abnormalities are often distinctive: prolongation of the QT interval, prominent U waves, and broad, large T waves with or without reversed polarity. Other wave form abnormalities seen with neurologic disease are ST depression (or elevation?) and flattened T waves, both of which may be erroneously attributed to organic heart disease, electrolyte disorders, or drug effects.

A strong association exists between the incidence of many arrhythmias and the presence of central nervous system disease. Arrhythmias range from sinus bradycardia and tachycardia to ectopic rhythms, to AV nodal blocks, with no single arrhythmia found to be characteristic. In a study of 135 patients with stroke, Reinstein et al observed cardiac arrhythmias in 61% during the first three days after onset.

The mechanism by which neurologic disease alters both rhythm and ECG wave forms has not been fully defined. The effect of acetylcholine has been implicated, as has been the increased autonomic activity initiated in the hypothalamus and mediated through the excessive secretion of catecholamines. Evidence for this concept is based largely on animal experiments, observing the myocardial effects of electrical activation of brain centers and the effects of catecholamine injections.

## SELECTED READINGS

Goldman MR, Rogers EL, Rogers MC: Subarachnoid hemorrhage—association with unusual electrocardiographic changes. *JAMA* 234:957–958, 1975.

Hall RE, Sybers HD, Greenhoot JH, et al: Myocardial alterations following hypothalamic stimulation in the intact conscious dog. *Am Heart J* 88:770–776, 1974.

Hammer WJ, Luessenhop AJ, Weintraub AM: Observations on the electrocardiographic changes associated with subarachnoid hemorrhage with special reference to their genesis. *Am J Med* 59:427–433, 1975.

Reinstein L, et al: Cardiac monitoring of the acute stroke patient. *Arch Phys Med Rehabil* 53:311, 1972.

## NUMBER 39 *Three's Company* Stephen P. Glasser, Pamela I. Clark

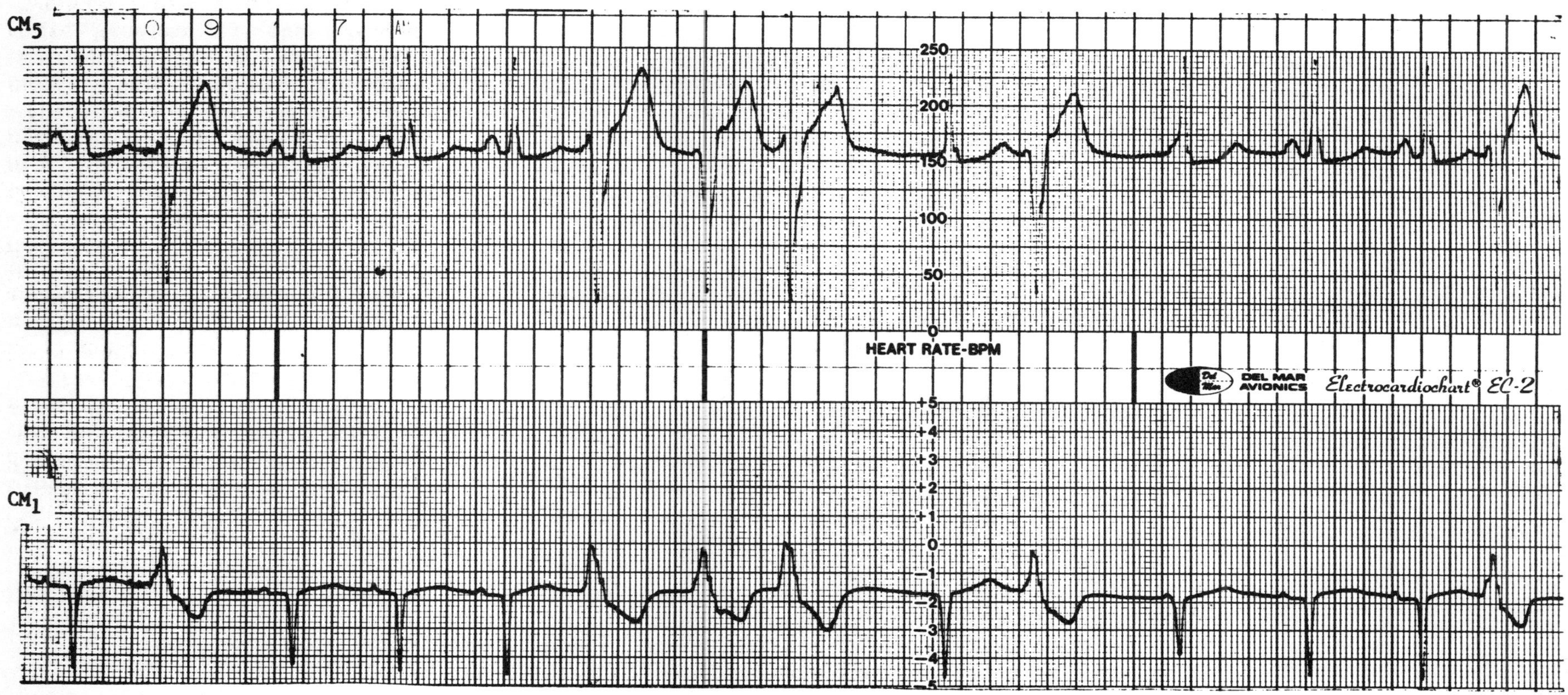


**Figure 39** A 38-year-old man suffered an inferior-wall, myocardial infarction. His convalescence was uncomplicated, and two weeks' postinfarction he was completely ambulatory without symptoms. Physical examination revealed an $S_4$ but was otherwise normal, and resting ECG showed only the residual changes of an inferior infarction. Ambulatory (Holter) monitoring was obtained by his private physician as a routine procedure prior to discharge.

# NUMBER 39 *Three's Company* Stephen P. Glasser, Pamela I. Clark

## ELUCIDATION

**Diagnosis—***Ventricular tachycardia*

The ambulatory ECG record revealed rare VPBs, but also one three-beat salvo of asymptomatic ventricular tachycardia as shown. Note that the salvo is initiated by a late VPB.

## DISCUSSION

Ventricular ectopy occurs frequently in patients with coronary disease and its prognostic significance has been the subject of increasing interest. Since the advent of acute coronary care and, recently, of ambulatory (Holter) monitoring, it has become apparent that paroxysmal ventricular tachycardia (PVT) in acute or recent myocardial infarction is not an uncommon rhythm disturbance. Although not fully elucidated, it has been generally assumed that significant ventricular arrhythmia in the patient after infarction carried a poor prognosis with regard to survival. Because of this, ambulatory monitoring has been recommended by some as part of the predischarge "routine" following myocardial infarction.

DeSoyza et al found that PVT noted during the acute phase of myocardial infarction correlated poorly with subsequent mortality. Of eight patients who died of cardiac causes after discharge, only one had PVT during the initial 24 hours of myocardial infarction. Of the 38 patients who survived an average of 19 months postinfarction, 17 had PVT during the initial 24 hours of their illness. The incidence of ventricular arrhythmia at the time of hospital discharge was similar to another report. This incidence was also similar to that found in a group of asymptomatic ambulatory men described by Hinkle. Anderson et al specifically evaluated a group of 66 patients who survived acute myocardial infarction and were subsequently found to have at least one run of ventricular tachycardia (VT) in the follow-up period—a subset of patients exemplified by the patient presented in this report. Life table analysis of the survival of VT and control patients revealed a 48-month VT survival of 75% compared with 87% in the control group. Their conclusion was that the occurrence of VT in the posthospital phase of myocardial infarction, while associated with a lower survival rate, does not indicate as much danger as is generally assumed.

An additional feature of this patient's arrhythmia is the initiation of VT after a long coupling interval. There has been great interest in the concept that VPBs with short coupling intervals are most likely to precipitate VT. However, deSoyza et al have reported that the majority of postinfarction patients with VT had VPBs with long coupling intervals and Ambos et al confirmed those findings by demonstrating that late VPBs initiated 85% of the episodes of VT in their study of 25 patients.

## SELECTED READINGS


Ambos HD, Roberts R, Low CW, et al: Late ectopic ventricular beats: precipitants of repetitive dysrhythmia. *Circulation* 53-54 (suppl II)II-8, 1976.

Anderson KP, DeCamilla J, Moss AJ: Clinical significance of ventricular tachycardia (3 beats or longer) detected during ambulatory monitoring after myocardial infarction. *Circulation* 57(5):890–897, 1978.

deSoyza N, Bennett FA, Murphy ML, et al: The relationship of paroxysmal ventricular tachycardia complicating the acute phase and ventricular arrhythmia during the late hospital phase of myocardial infarction to long-term survival. *Am J Med* 64:377–381, 1978.

deSoyza N, et al: Ectopic ventricular prematurity and its relationship to ventricular tachycardia in acute myocardial infarction in man. *Circulation* 50:529, 1974.

Hinkle LA, et al: The frequency of asymptomatic disturbances of cardiac rhythm and conduction in middle-aged men. *Am J Cardiol* 24:629, 1969.

Moss AJ, et al: Ventricular arrhythmias three weeks after myocardial infarction. *Ann Intern Med* 75:937, 1971.

## NUMBER 40 *Double Trouble* Stephen P. Glasser, Pamela I. Clark

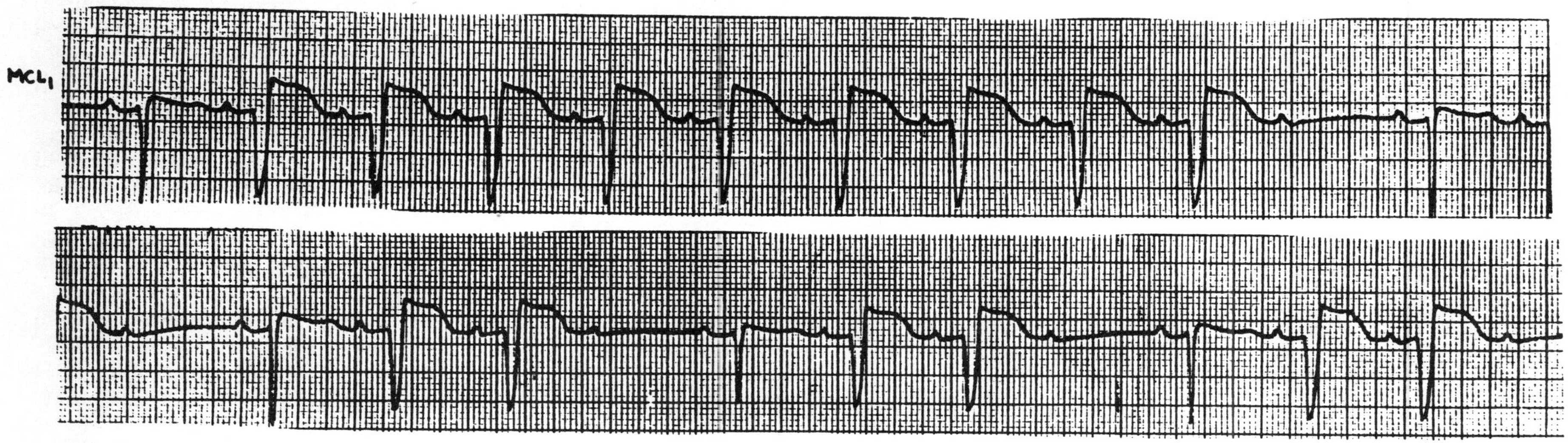


**Figure 40** The patient whose ECG is shown here was a 62-year-old man with dizzy spells.

# NUMBER 40 *Double Trouble* Stephen P. Glasser, Pamela I. Clark

## ELUCIDATION

The $MCL_1$ lead demonstrates constant PR and PP intervals with some P waves that are not conducted (dropped). In addition, the bottom strip shows groups of three ventricular complexes with gradual prolongation of the intraventricular conduction time. This ECG then demonstrates two conduction system problems: Mobitz II second degree AV block and Wenckebach block in the left bundle branch system.

## DISCUSSION

Two varieties of second degree atrioventricular (AV) block are described. In the first (Mobitz I block) there is progressive lengthening of the PR interval until a dropped beat occurs. The term Wenckebach periodicity is used to describe this sequence. In the other variety of second-degree block (Mobitz II block) dropped beats are not preceded by PR lengthening. Mobitz I block generally occurs because of disease of the AV node, while Mobitz II block is generally a result of block in both bundle branch systems.

Since Wenckebach first described the periodic block which follows progressive prolongation of the PR interval, several authors have pointed out that such a phenomenon has also been observed in the bundle branches. Here, groups of beats demonstrate progressive lengthening in the degree of bundle branch block up to the complete bundle branch block beat which then terminates the period. This sequence should not be surprising since electrograms recording the potentials of specific components of the conduction system in situ have confirmed the hypothesis suggested by experimental studies that most of the electrophysiologic properties of the system are common to all its components.

Wenckebach bundle branch block has been described in the right bundle, left bundle, and left anterior fascicle, and probably occurs more frequently than previously suspected. Only an awareness of its occurrence and accurate diagnostic criteria will reveal its true frequency and prognostic implications.

## SELECTED READINGS

Cristal N, Ho W: Second degree block within the bundle branches. *Chest* 66:57–60, 1974.

Friedberg HD, Schamroth L: The Wenckebach phenomenon in left bundle branch block. *Am J Cardiol* 24:591–594, 1969.

Mangiola S: Intermittent left anterior hemiblock with Wenckebach phenomenon. *Am J Cardiol* 30:892–895, 1972.

Rosenbaum MB, Nau GJ, Levi RJ, et al: Wenckebach periods in the bundle branches. *Circulation* 40:79–86, 1969.

## NUMBER 41 *Twenty-four Hours with the Happy Holter* Stephen P. Glasser, Pamela I. Clark

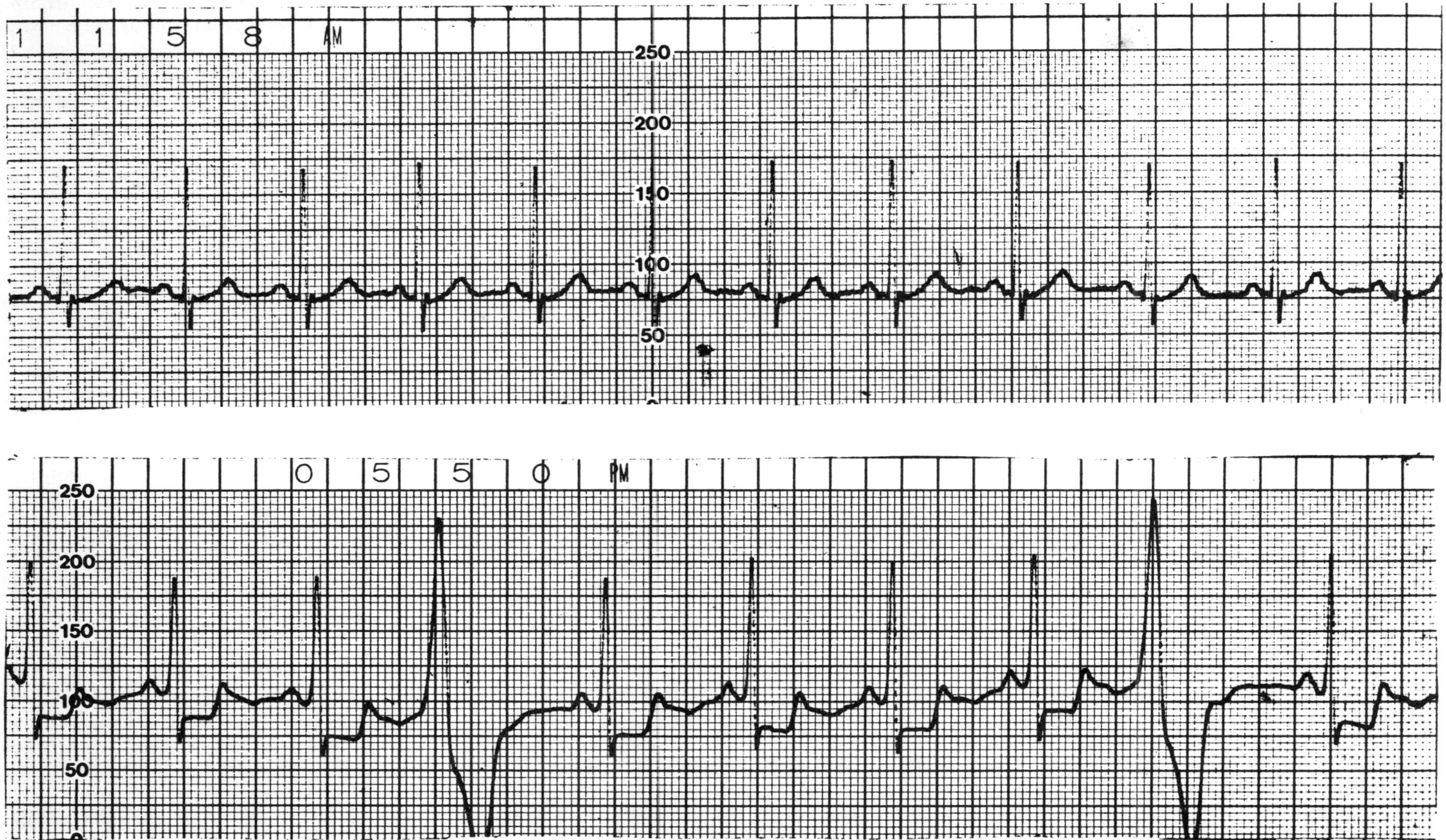


**Figure 41** A 68-year-old man had six months of progressive angina pectoris. With medical treatment, he developed chronic stable angina occurring two to four times per week. A treadmill exercise test was markedly positive. Ambulatory (Holter) monitoring was performed in order to investigate the occurrence of symptomatic and asymptomatic ischemic episodes.

# NUMBER 41 *Twenty-four Hours with the Happy Holter* Stephen P. Glasser, Pamela I. Clark

## ELUCIDATION

**Diagnosis**—*Ischemic S-T depression*

The figure demonstrates two representative strips from the patient's ambulatory ECG recording. The top strip recorded at 11:58 AM demonstrates sinus rhythm at a rate of 94 beats per minute (bpm) and normal S-T segments. The bottom strip recorded at 5:50 PM also shows sinus rhythm, but the rate is slower (75 bpm) and marked S-T segment depression (4 mm) is present. Two ventricular premature beats are also noted. Analysis of his diary revealed no symptoms during this episode of S-T depression, but similar episodes of S-T depression at faster heart rates were associated with classic angina.

## DISCUSSION

Ambulatory monitoring has gained wide acceptance for the detection of arrhythmias and conduction disturbances, but only limited acceptance for the evaluation of S-T segments. This limited acceptance was based upon the inadequate frequency response characteristic of the early recording systems (resulting in poor reproduction of the low frequency S-T segment) as well as the effects of postural and physiologic changes on the S-T segment. The lack of amplitude standardization also suggested that clinical application might prove unreliable.

In spite of these early reservations, a number of studies have emerged that suggest that a renewed interest in the S-T segment response during ambulatory monitoring is warranted. Two studies compare the S-T segment response occurring during ambulatory monitoring with that of the exercise test and demonstrate that the two are comparable. Stern and Tzivoni evaluated the presence and absence of S-T changes during ambulatory monitoring and related this to angiographically determined coronary anatomy demonstrating a sensitivity of 91% and specificity of 78%. These authors also indicated that ambulatory S-T changes had a high predictive value for future cardiac morbid events.

Ambulatory monitoring has revealed that patients with coronary disease may manifest ischemic S-T depression during angina as well as without symptoms (as seen in the patient presented). Commonly, nonanginal S-T depression occurs at lower heart rates than those observed with typical angina or produced during exercise testing. The meaning of these observations is not yet fully known.

## SELECTED READINGS


Kennedy HL, Caralis DG: Ambulatory electrocardiography—a clinical perspective. *Ann Intern Med* 87:729–739, 1977.

Kennedy HL: Detection of ST-segment depression with Holter system. *Ambulatory/electrocardiology* 1:11–12, 1977.

O'Rourke RA, Ross J: Ambulatory electrocardiographic monitoring to detect ischemic heart disease. *Ann Inter Med* 81:695–696, 1974.

Schang SJ, Pepine CJ: Transient asymptomatic S-T segment depression during daily activity. *Am J Cardiol* 39:396–402, 1977.

Stern S, Tzivoni D: Early detection of silent ischaemic heart disease by 24-hour electrocardiographic monitoring of active subjects. *Br Heart J* 36:481–486, 1974.

Wolf E, Tzivoni D, Stern S: Comparison of exercise tests and 24-hour ambulatory electrocardiographic monitoring in detection of ST-T changes. *Br Heart J* 36:90–95, 1977.

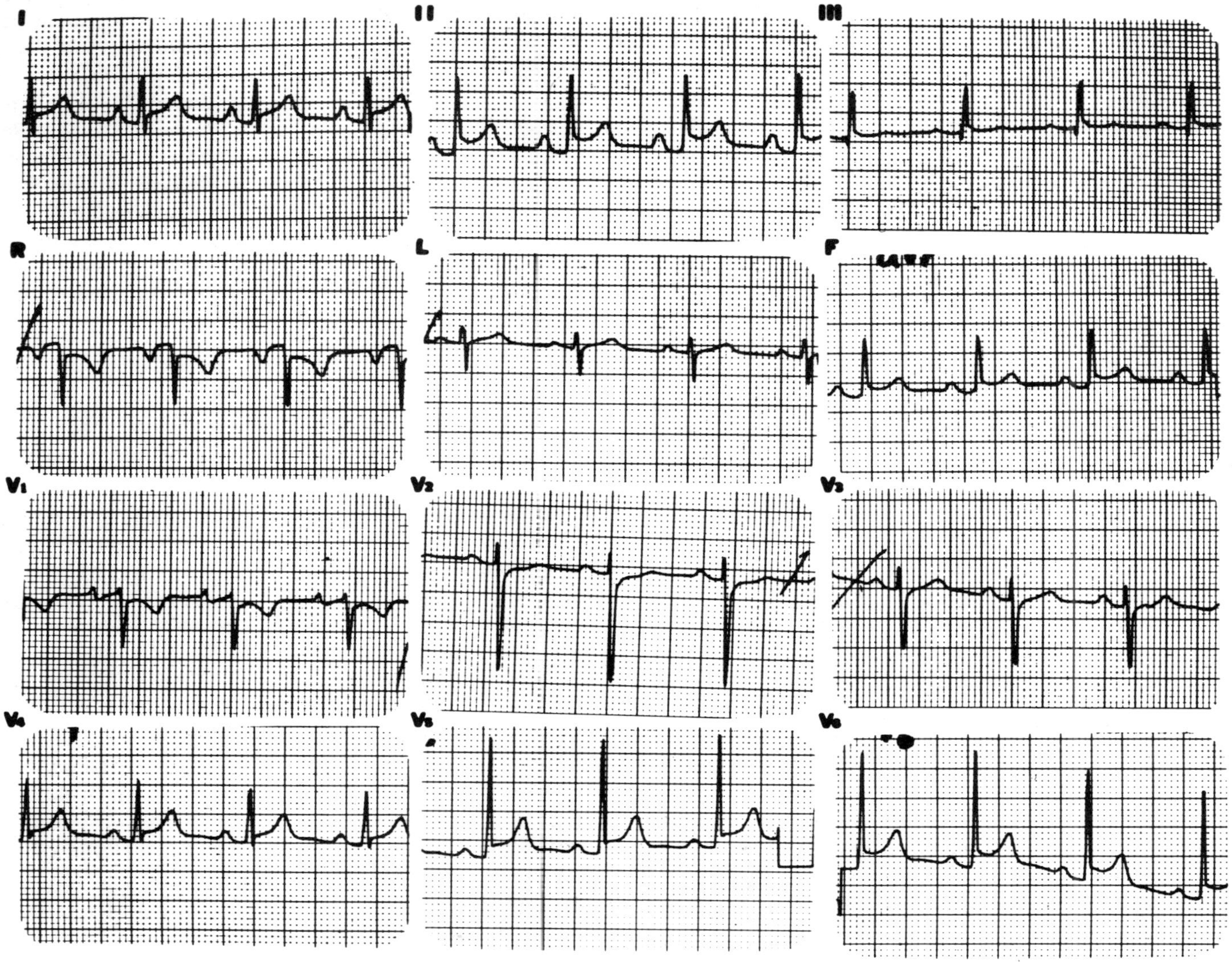


**Figure 42** The patient whose electrocardiogram is shown was a 21-year-old man with chest pain. Physical examination was normal.

# NUMBER 42 *Atrial Injury Current* Stephen P. Glasser

## ELUCIDATION

The ECG demonstrates ST-segment elevation in leads I, II, III, aVF, $V_4$, $V_5$, and $V_6$. This entails a differential diagnosis of acute myocardial infarction, pericarditis, and the pattern of early repolarization. The changes are too diffuse for acute myocardial infarction, and there is no reciprocal ST segment depression (aVR and, to a lesser extent, $V_1$ simulate intracavitary leads. Therefore, they would not be expected to show ST-segment elevation in pericarditis). This tracing could represent an early repolarization pattern (a normal variant not uncommon in young blacks). The tip-off that this was indeed pericarditis is the current of injury in the repolarization of the P wave (the so-called S-Ta segment abnormalities).

## DISCUSSION

One might suspect that the current of injury in atrial pericarditis would be directed toward the right shoulder and, indeed, in our experience this has proved to be the case. Thus, one sees, as in this tracing, an elevated S-Ta segment most prominently in aVR.

The other typical ECG changes of pericarditis are, of course, evolutionary. Following the RS-T elevation there are flattening and then inversion of the T waves as the RS-T elevation returns to baseline. The patient subsequently presented with this evolutionary change after developing a classic three-component pericardial friction rub due to viral pericarditis.

Atrial repolarization abnormalities might well be anticipated in pericarditis overlying the atrial myocardium, since ventricular repolarization abnormalities occur in pericarditis overlying the ventricular myocardium. Furthermore, it would be expected that S-Ta segment abnormalities would be a common accompaniment, and yet these changes have been rarely commented upon. Atrial arrhythmias, morphologic P-wave changes, and S-Ta segment abnormalities are the generally considered electrocardiographic hallmarks of atrial injury. S-Ta segment abnormalities have been associated with atrial abscesses, coronary arteritis, coronary arteriosclerosis, congenital anomalies of the coronary vessels, cardiac catheterization, and atrial infarction.

An atrial injury current originating at the epicardial surface of the atria should result in a net vector toward lead aVR. This would result in S-Ta segment elevation in that lead and S-Ta segment depressions in other leads. Tranchesi et al's review article on atrial repolarization abnormalities in general discusses a case of pericarditis with just such changes. Once we started to look for this change, we found it to be rather common. We believe that this change could provide a valuable clue in the diagnosis of acute pericarditis in general, and in certain specific instances it may be of additional value. Thus, in patients with an enlarging cardiac silhouette, S-Ta segment changes might aid in differentiating pericarditis from primary myocardial disease. Because of early repolarization, Feinstein and Spagnuolo do not include ventricular S-Ta segment elevation as a diagnostic criterion of pericarditis during acute rheumatic fever.

Abramson et al were perhaps the first to study critically the electrical activity of the atria. Cauterization of the atrial wall in dogs resulted in consistent S-Ta segment changes. Changes in P-wave morphology also occurred but to a lesser extent. Stewart and Manning, in analyzing the EKGs of 500 normal airmen, found only slight depression of the PR segment not exceeding 0.5 mm; Shipley and Hallaran found 55% of 200 normal men had S-Ta segment depression in lead I but none exceeded 0.8 mm. Only two showed S-Ta segment elevation and they were each less than 0.4 mm. Gross found some correlation of S-Ta segment depression and heart rate, but not greater than 1.0 mm, and usually up to 0.50 mm. On the other hand, Scherf and Schaffer in their analysis of the ECG with exercise did not note S-Ta segment changes.

We would then agree with Young and Koenig that it is highly probable that any ECG in which S-Ta segment depression of more than 0.8 mm or elevation more than 0.5 mm may be considered strongly suggestive of atrial damage. Finally, several well documented cases of atrial infarction and an analysis of electrocardiographic changes during cardiac surgery demonstrate that atrial injury can result in S-Ta segment changes.

Thus, Spodick in a review article on the differential diagnosis of acute pericarditis states as one of the typical ECG changes of pericarditis that "the PR segment frequently becomes depressed with respect to the T and P interval, best seen in lead II and probably due to atrial pericarditis." We would differ only in that we feel lead aVR is best analyzed.

## SELECTED READINGS


Abramson DI, Fenichel NM, Shookhoff C: A study of electrical activity in the auricles. *Am Heart J* 15:471, 1938.

Cushing EH, et al: Infarction of the cardiac auricles (atria). *Br Heart J* 4:17, 1942.

Dicosky C, Zimmerman HA: Atrial injury. *J Electrocardiol* 2:51, 1969.

Di Ielsi AJ, Pinsky HA, Eynon HK: Auricular infarction: report of two cases. *Ann Intern Med* 36:640, 1952.

Feinstein AR, Spagnuolo M: Clinical patterns of acute rheumatic fever. *Medicine* 41:279, 1962.

Friedberg CK: *Diseases of the Heart.* Philadelphia, WB Saunders Company, 1966, p 943.

Gross D: The auricular T wave and its correlation to the cardiac rate and to the P wave. *Am Heart J* 50:24, 1955.

Jaruszewski EJ, Hellerstein HK, Feil H: Electrocardiographic studies during cardiac surgery. *Circulation* 7:175, 1953.

Robert JT, Loube SD: Congenital single coronary artery in men. *Am Heart J* 34:188, 1947.

Scherf D, Schaffer AI: The electrocardiographic exercise test. *Am Heart J* 43:927, 1952.

Shipley R, Hallaran W: The four lead electrocardiogram in 200 normal men and women. *Am Heart J* 11:325, 1936.

Spodick DH: Differential diagnosis of acute pericarditis. *Prog Cardiovasc Dis* 14:192, 1971.

Stewart LB, Manning GW: A detailed analysis of the electrocardiograms of 500 RCAF aircrew. *Am Heart J* 27:502, 1944.

Tranchesi J, Adelardi V, de Oliveira JM: Atrial repolarization: its importance in clinical electrocardiography. *Circulation* 22:635, 1960.

Wilson JL, Knudson KP: Infarction of the cardiac atria. *N Engl J Med* 251:559, 1954.

Young EW, Koenig A: Auricular infarction. *Am Heart J* 28:287, 1944.

## NUMBER 43 *Noctecardia* Karen Bowyer, Stephen P. Glasser

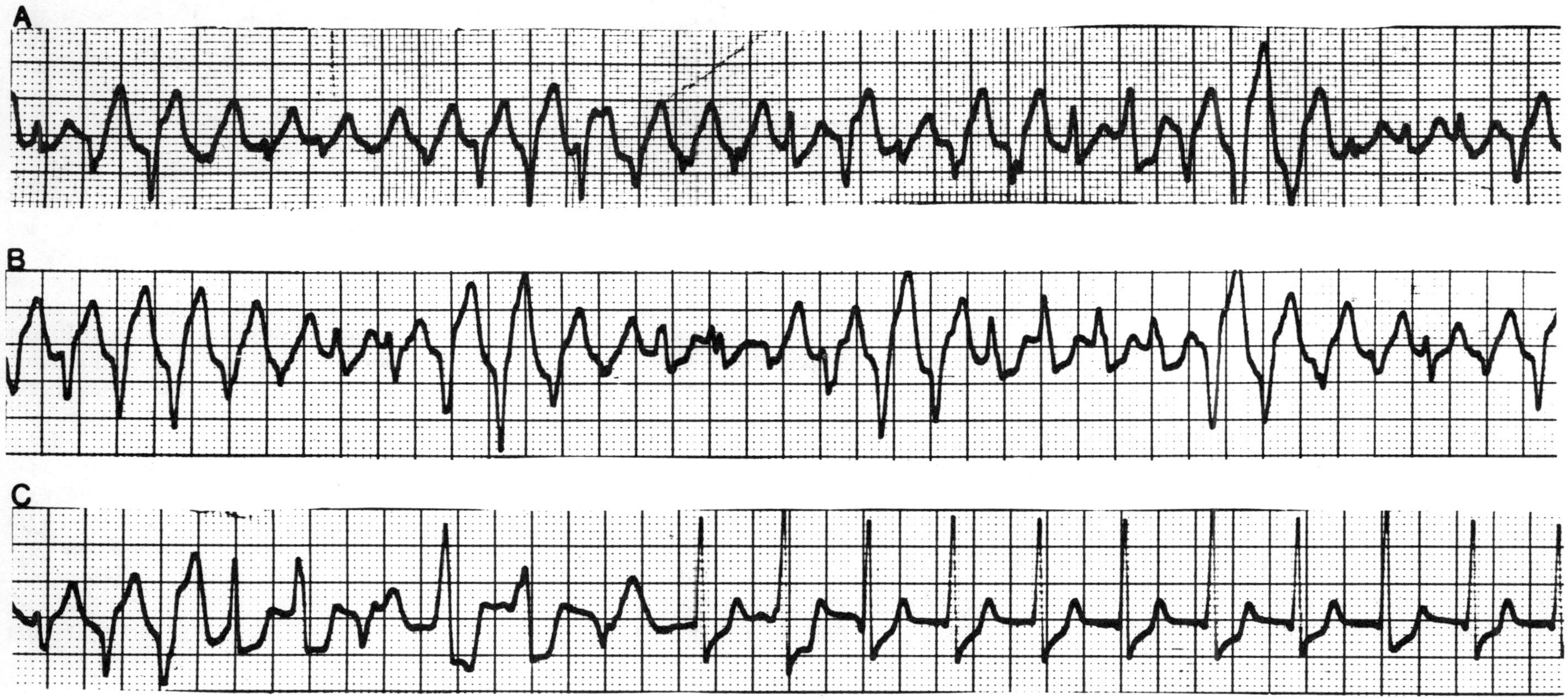


**Figure 43** A 17-year-old man ingested 28 Noctec (chloral hydrate) capsules four hours prior to admission. On arrival in the emergency room, he was comatose and the ECG shown (panel A) was obtained. An endotracheal tube was placed for ventilatory support and gastric lavage was performed. Lidocaine (75-mg IV bolus) followed by an intravenous drip of 5 mg/min resulted in little improvement (panel B). Propranolol (1 mg IV), however, resulted in stabilization of the rhythm (panel C), and within 24 hours he was awake, alert, and in sinus rhythm. He was discharged to psychiatric care three days later.

# NUMBER 43 *Noctecardia* Karen Bowyer, Stephen P. Glasser

## ELUCIDATION

Panels A and B demonstrate multiform ventricular tachycardia. Midway through panel C (moments after the administration of IV propranolol) the rhythm converts to a junctional tachycardia.

## DISCUSSION

Several cases have been reported of cardiac arrhythmias (mainly multiform ventricular tachycardia and junctional tachycardia) occurring in adult patients without underlying heart disease following chloral hydrate overdosage of greater than 10 g. Chloral hydrate has been shown to shorten the refractory period and depress contractility of the myocardium with large doses, but seems reasonably safe in therapeutic doses since it has been used safely for sedation even in patients with heart disease.

Of the cases of chloral hydrate overdosage associated with arrhythmia, several are worthy of comment. DiGiovanni reported a case of refractory ventricular arrhythmia in which lidocaine produced only temporary rhythm control. Finally, alprenolol (5 mg IV) was administered with resultant marked stabilization of rhythm. In the case reported by Marshall, procinolol was used successfully for ventricular tachycardia which occurred following chloral hydrate overdosage. In the patient presented here, ventricular arrhythmia also proved refractory to lidocaine but responded immediately to intravenous propranolol.

The explanation for the favorable response to propranolol of dysrhythmias secondary to chloral hydrate is speculative. Marshall believed that chloral hydrate may sensitize the myocardium to circulating catecholamines in the same way that chloroform does. Regardless, it appears that lidocaine is the drug often used in the treatment of ventricular arrhythmias secondary to excessive chloral hydrate intake. But, of the five patients so treated, lidocaine was successful for arrhythmia control in only one. This is compared to the three instances in which propranolol was utilized, and it was immediately successful in each. Certainly, a larger series of cases would be necessary to establish the appropriate treatment regimen for ventricular arrhythmias occurring in the setting of chloral hydrate overdosage, but our review suggests that propranolol should be given high consideration if contraindications for its use are not present.

## SELECTED READINGS


Bowyer K, Glasser SP: Chloral hydrate and cardiac arrhythmias. Noctecardia case report and review of the literature. *Chest* (in press)

DiGiovanni AJ: Reversal of chloral hydrate associated cardiac arrhythmia by a beta-adrenergic blocking agent. *Anesthesiology* 31(1):93, 1969.

Gleich G, Morgan E, Vaules D: Esophageal stricture following chloral hydrate poisoning. *JAMA* 201:266, 1967.

Gustafson A, Swenson S, Ugander L: Arrhythmias in chloral hydrate poisoning. *Acta Med Scand* 201:227, 1977.

Malach M, Berman N: Furosemide and chloral hydrate. *JAMA* 232:638, 1975.

Marshall AJ: Cardiac arrhythmias caused by chloral hydrate. *Br Med J* 2:994, 1977.

Muller SA, Fisch C: Cardiac arrhythmia due to use of chloral hydrate. *J Indiana State Med Assoc* 49:38, 1956.

Nordenberg A, Delisle G, Izukana T: Cardiac arrhythmia in a child due to chloral hydrate ingestion. *Pediatrics* 47:134, 1971.

Sharpless SK: In Goodman LS, Gilman A (eds): *The Pharmacological Basis of Therapeutics.* London, Macmillan Publishers Ltd, 1970, p 123.

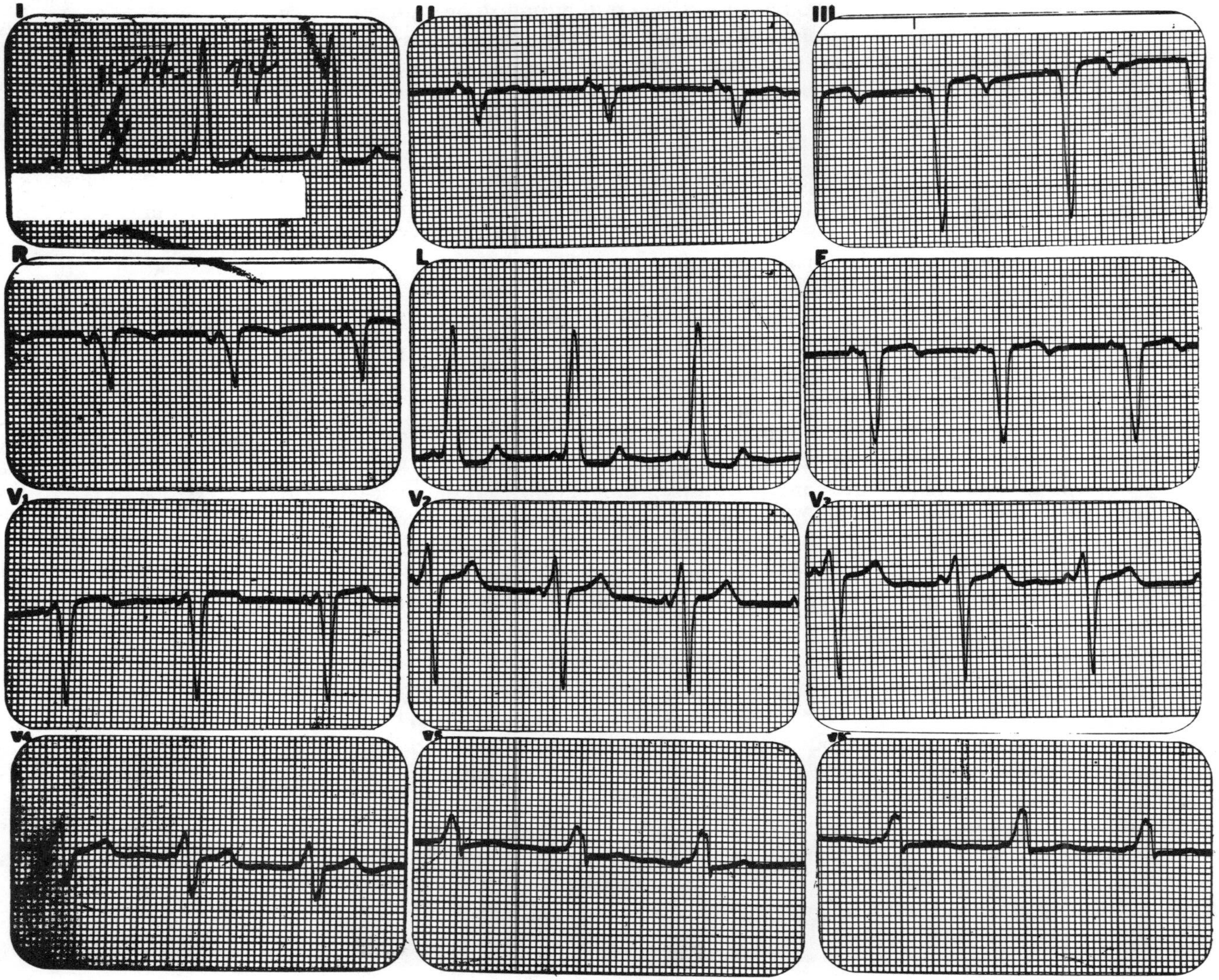


**Figure 44** This ECG was obtained from a 40-year-old man with a history of palpitations during which vague chest discomfort was experienced. No prior ECGs were available for comparison.

# NUMBER 44 *The Pre-Excitation Syndromes* Stephen P. Glasser

## ELUCIDATION

The PR interval is 0.08 second with essentially no PR segment. The QRS complex is widened to 0.12 second with the lengthening occurring in the initial segments of the QRS complex. Secondary ST-segment and T-wave changes are present. These findings are diagnostic of the Wolff-Parkinson-White (WPW) syndrome. This particular tracing mimics an inferior wall myocardial infarction.

## DISCUSSION

The original description of the WPW syndrome in 1930 characterized it as "bundle branch block with a short PR interval in healthy young people prone to paroxysmal tachycardia." Since then, much has been written, much new knowledge revealed, and much confusion in terminology has resulted. The basic features of the classical WPW syndrome consist of a PR interval not exceeding 0.12 second, a delta wave (as manifested by the initial deformity of the QRS complex), and a QRS width of 0.12 second or longer. However, variants of the WPW syndrome have now been described and are collectively termed the pre-excitation syndromes.

Pre-excitation exists if, in relation to atrial events, the whole or some part of the ventricular muscle is activated earlier by the impulse conducted through the aberrant pathway than would be expected if the impulse reached the ventricles by way of the normal conduction system. There have now been enough recent studies of the anatomy of accessory pathways between the atria and ventricles in association with electrophysiologic studies and epicardial mapping which indicate that ventricular pre-excitation almost certainly results from accessory atrioventricular bypass tracts short-circuiting the normal AV conduction pathway. This then causes an abbreviation of the PR interval and widening of the QRS duration. Three such bypass tracts have been described: 1) Kent bundles, which result in the classical and most common form of WPW; 2) Mahaim fibers, which result in the variant of normal PR interval with abnormal QRS; and 3) James and Mahaim fibers. The James bypass results in the abbreviated PR interval but with QRS complexes of normal duration (ie, the LGL syndrome), while the Mahaim tract results in the widening QRS complex.

Other examples of the variants include: 1) a PR interval less than 0.12 second with a small delta wave resulting in a QRS duration of 0.10 to 0.12 second; and 2) the PR interval measuring greater than 0.12 second but with the other features of WPW.

If one accepts the view that the importance of the WPW syndrome lies in the propensity to tachycardia, then all of these anatomic modalities are of equal clinical significance, fulfilling prerequisites for initiation of reciprocating tachycardias, that is, two pathways with unequal conduction velocity permit the initiating impulse to set up a circus pathway. Of additional importance, however, is the fact that the conduction abnormality may mimic other ECG changes, or otherwise obscure diagnostic findings. Thus, once WPW syndrome is recognized, no further comments can be made regarding ventricular hypertrophy, infarct patterns, or abnormalities of ventricular depolarization or repolarization.

No treatment is indicated for the isolated abnormality; treatment of supraventricular arrhythmias is similar to that which is given in the absence of the WPW syndrome. There is one note of caution, and that is in the case of atrial fibrillation or flutter when the QRS complexes display the features of WPW, indicating that antegrade conduction proceeds through the accessory pathway and not across the AV node. Even toxic doses of digitalis may not slow the ventricular rate in such cases and might even worsen the arrhythmia.

## SELECTED READINGS


Castellanos A, Lemberg L, Claxton BW: Wolff-Parkinson-White syndrome: generalities. *Chest* 65:307–322, 1974.

Durrer D, Schuilenburg RM, Wellens HJJ: Pre-excitation revisited. *Am J Cardiol* 25:690–697, 1970.

Massumi RA, Mason DT, Vera A, et al: The Wolff-Parkinson-White syndrome. *Postgrad Med* 53:49–57, 1973.

Moore EN, Spear JF, Boineau JP: Recent electrophysiologic studies on the Wolff-Parkinson-White syndrome. *N Engl J Med* 289:956–963, 1973.

Narula OS: Wolf-Parkinson-White syndrome. *Circulation* 47:872–886, 1973.

# NUMBER 45 *The Pause That Refreshes*

Stephen P. Glasser, Pamela I. Clark

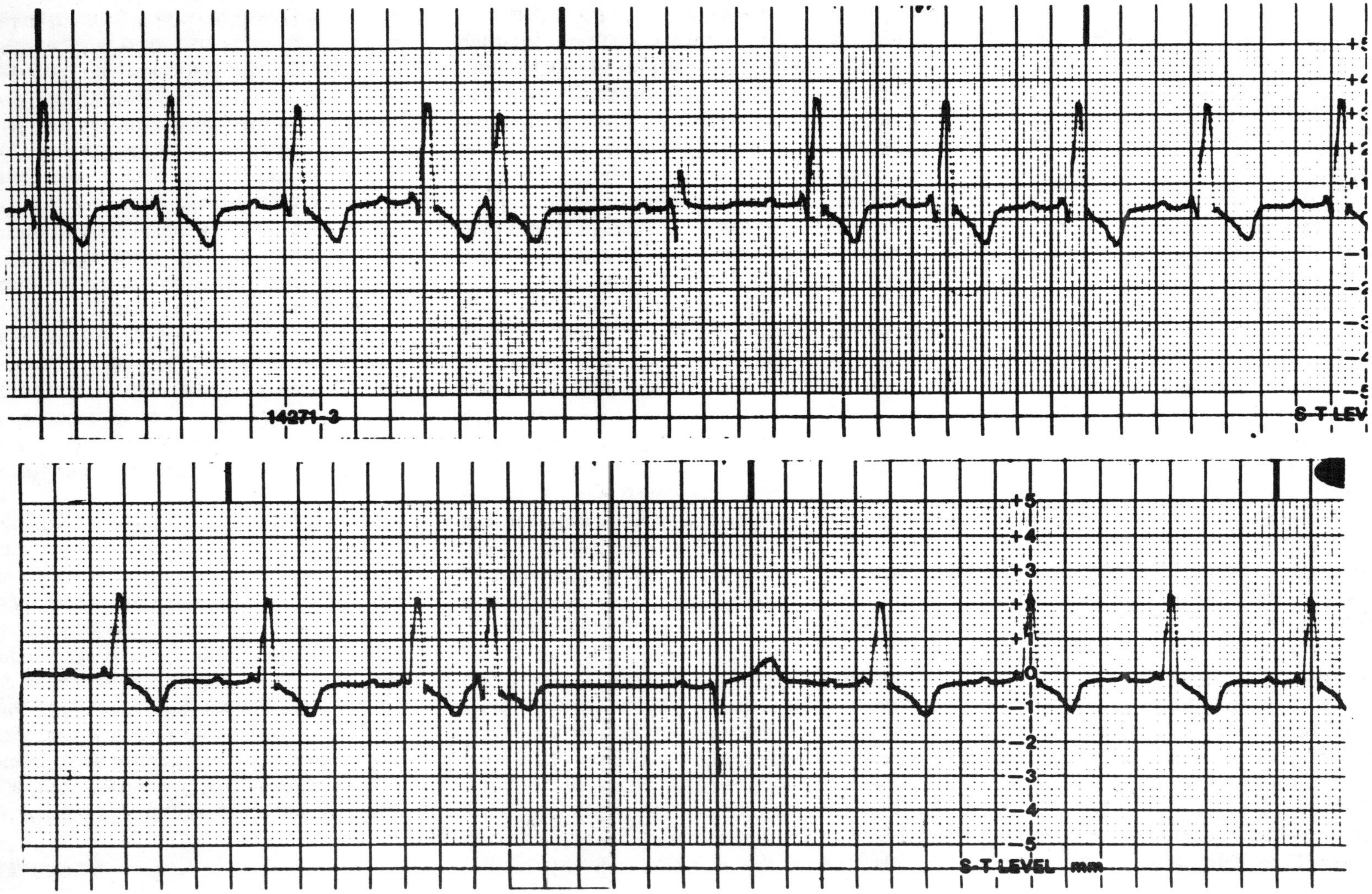


**Figure 45** A 63-year-old man with palpitations was referred for ambulatory monitoring. His physical examination was normal except for mild hypertension controlled by daily hydrochlorothiazide. His resting electrocardiogram demonstrated a complete right bundle branch block, known to be present for at least five years. The monitoring strips are not continuous, and are taken from the modified $V_1$ lead.

# NUMBER 45 *The Pause That Refreshes*

Stephen P. Glasser, Pamela I. Clark

## ELUCIDATION

The dominant rhythm is sinus with right bundle branch block (RBBB). In both the top and bottom strips premature junctional beats occur, followed by pauses of 1040 msec (top strip) and 1360 msec (bottom strip). In the top strip the pause is terminated by a sinus beat conducted with an incomplete RBBB; but in the bottom strip the pause is terminated by a normally conducted, narrow QRS beat. This suggests that the RBBB is a rate-related phenomenon.

## DISCUSSION

Intermittent bundle branch block is thought to be caused by hypopolarization, slow diastolic depolarization, a shift of the action potential threshold closer to zero or, most commonly in the absence of acute myocardial injury, prolongation of recovery in one or more of the bundle branches. The refractory period of each conduction fascicle is directly proportional to the preceding cycle length. Thus, at sufficiently high heart rates, impulses reach the affected bundle branch during the prolonged refractory period, and slowed conduction or block results. Below the critical rate, impulses reach the fascicles after recovery is completed, and conduction is normal. Sometimes the critical rate is such that only during exercise will the conduction defect become manifest; while sometimes normal conduction will be seen only when the rate is unusually slow (eg, the case shown here).

Bundle branch block which develops as the heart rate accelerates is termed rate-dependent bundle branch block, and the heart rate at which intraventricular conduction changes is termed the critical rate. The critical heart rate has been shown experimentally and clinically often to be lower for return to normal conduction than for the initiation of bundle branch block.

Prolongation of refractory periods occurs primarily in older individuals and in diseased hearts. Rate-dependent left bundle branch block, at relatively low heart rates (130 beats per minute and less) generally implies cardiac abnormality, organic disease, functional alteration, or drug effects. Intermittent left bundle branch block tends eventually to become fixed and permanent. This apparently is less true for rate-dependent RBBB, perhaps because normally the right bundle branch has a longer refractory period than the remainder of the conduction system.

Persons with intermittent left bundle branch block frequently have abnormal repolarization patterns after returning to normal intraventricular conduction. Engel and coworkers and Denes et al reported persistent symmetrical, deeply inverted precordial T waves with return of narrow QRS conduction following temporary left bundle branch block. The pattern was seen in 72% of Engel's 33 patients and in 83% of Denes's 23 patients, and was similar to the abnormal repolarization patterns seen with interruption of artificial ventricular pacing. Complicating further the ability to interpret S-T and T-wave abnormalities during narrow QRS conduction in the individuals with intermittent left bundle branch block is the possible persistence of some degree of incomplete left bundle branch block with secondary S-T and T-wave abnormalities. Abnormal ST-T waves are not expected to be seen in the lateral precordial leads of patients with right bundle branch block and, following conversion to normal conduction, abnormal ST-T wave shifts are not anticipated.

Bradycardia-dependent bundle branch block also occurs but is less common. In that case, normal conduction is the rule until the rate slows to a "critical" level and an intraventricular conduction defect occurs. Rarely, the conduction defect is manifest during normal daily activities, but with exercise tachycardia the QRS duration becomes normal.

## SELECTED READINGS

Bellet SP: *Clinical Disorders of the Heart Beat, ed 3.* Philadelphia, Lea & Febiger, 1971, pp 541–542.

Chatterjee K, Harris AM, Davies JG, et al: Electrocardiographic changes subsequent to artificial ventricular depolarization. *Br Heart J* 31:770, 1969.

Denes P, Pick A, Miller RH, et al: A characteristic precordial repolarization abnormality with intermittent left bundle-branch block. *Ann Intern Med* 89:55, 1978.

Engel TR, Shah R, DePodesta LA, et al: T-wave abnormalities of intermittent left bundle-branch block. *Ann Intern Med* 89:204, 1978.

Fisch C, Zipes DP, McHenry PL: Rate dependent aberrancy. *Circulation* 48:714, 1973.

Sandberg L: Electrocardiographic studies of cases where bundle-branch block develops during exercise tests. *Acta Med Scand* 169(suppl):78, 1961.

## NUMBER 46 *A Node of Caution* Stephen P. Glasser, Pamela I. Clark

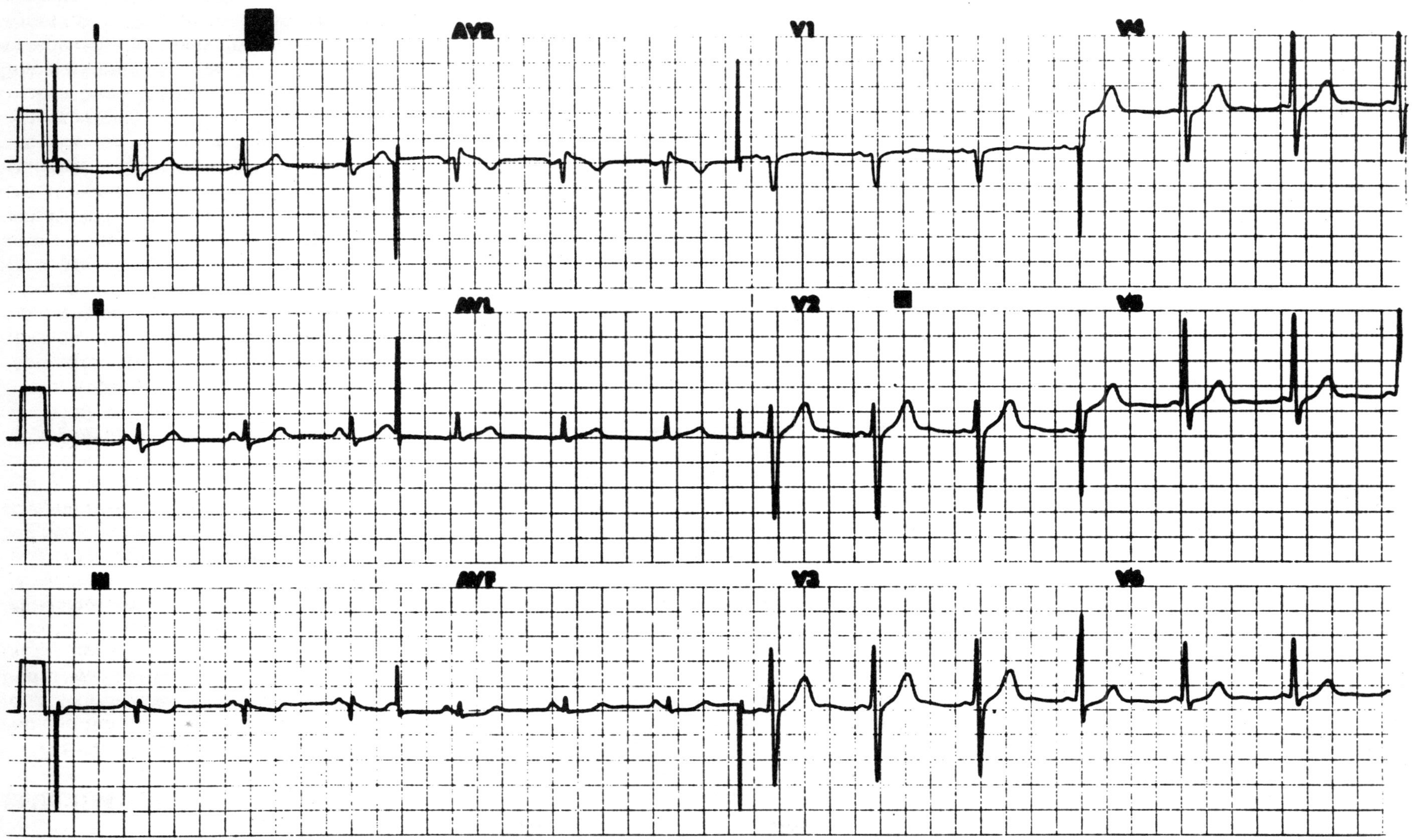


**Figure 46** The electrocardiogram is a routine preoperative tracing from a 52-year-old asymptomatic man about to undergo elective hernia surgery.

# NUMBER 46 *A Node of Caution* Stephen P. Glasser, Pamela I. Clark

## ELUCIDATION

A short PR interval (0.10 to 0.12 seconds) and normal QRS complex is present, and a form of accelerated atrioventricular conduction (LGL syndrome) is suggested.

## DISCUSSION

A short PR interval, wide QRS complex, and delta wave describes a form of accelerated atrioventricular conduction and is associated with a high incidence of supraventricular arrhythmia. It was described in 1930 and carries the eponym of the Wolff-Parkinson-White (WPW) syndrome.

In 1952 Lown, Ganong, and Levine[2] popularized the ECG syndrome (originally described by Clerc, Levy, and Critesco in 1938) consisting of a short PR interval, normal QRS complex, and paroxysmal tachycardias, which since has been proven to represent another form of accelerated atrioventricular conduction. It carries the eponym of its authors and is also known as the LGL syndrome. As with all eponyms, controversy as to the best terminology exists, but the common usage of the LGL syndrome persists.

Burch and Kimball first considered that the LGL syndrome could be due to the presence of an atrio—His bundle pathway. At present most authors consider that the short PR interval is due to the functional presence of an atrionodal bypass tract which was described by James in 1961. This type of bypass would then form the anatomical substrate for reentrant arrhythmias.

Electrophysiologic studies of the LGL syndrome and of subjects with short PR intervals without tachyarrhythmias further support the concept of an AV nodal bypass tract, but other explanations for a short PR interval (anatomically small AV node, a short or rapidly conducting intranodal pathway or isorhythmic AV dissociation) exist. When necessary, atrial pacing studies with simultaneous measurement of atrial-to-His bundle (A-H) conduction time is diagnostic. Thus, the normal response to atrial pacing is a prolongation of A-H time, a phenomenon that does not occur when a bypass tract exists. Also, in the setting of a bypass tract, pacing-induced atrial premature depolarizations may produce echo beats and sustained supraventricular tachycardia.

Variants of this syndrome (as in the WPW syndrome) have been described. For instance, the PR interval might be normal or long when intraatrial conduction time is prolonged. In the patient whose ECG is shown, an isolated short PR interval was noted on routine preoperative electrocardiography. Because he was asymptomatic, no further workup was recommended, and he underwent uneventful surgery.

## SELECTED READINGS


Burch GE, Kimball JL: Notes on the similarity of QRS complex configuration in Wolff Parkinson White syndrome. *Am Heart J* 32:560, 1946.

Clerc A, Levy R, Critesco C: A propos due raccour cissement permanent de e espace P-R de l'electrocardiogramme sans deformation du complex ventriculaire. *Arch Mal Coeur* 31:569, 1938.

Ferrer MI: New concepts relating to the preexcitation syndrome. *JAMA* 201:162, 1967.

Iannone LA: Electrophysiology of atrial pacing in patients with short PR interval, normal QRS complex. *Am Heart J* 89:74, 1975.

James TN: Morphology of the human atrioventricular node, with remarks pertinent to its electrophysiology. *Am Heart J* 62:756, 1961.

Lown B, Ganong WF, Levine SA: The syndrome of short P-R interval, normal QRS complex and paroxysmal rapid heart action. *Circulation* 5:693, 1952.

Wolff L, Parkinson J, White PD: Bundle-branch block with short P-R interval in healthy young people prone to paroxysmal tachycardia. *Am Heart J* 5:685, 1930.

## NUMBER 47 *Run Silent, Run Deep* Stephen P. Glasser, Pamela I. Clark

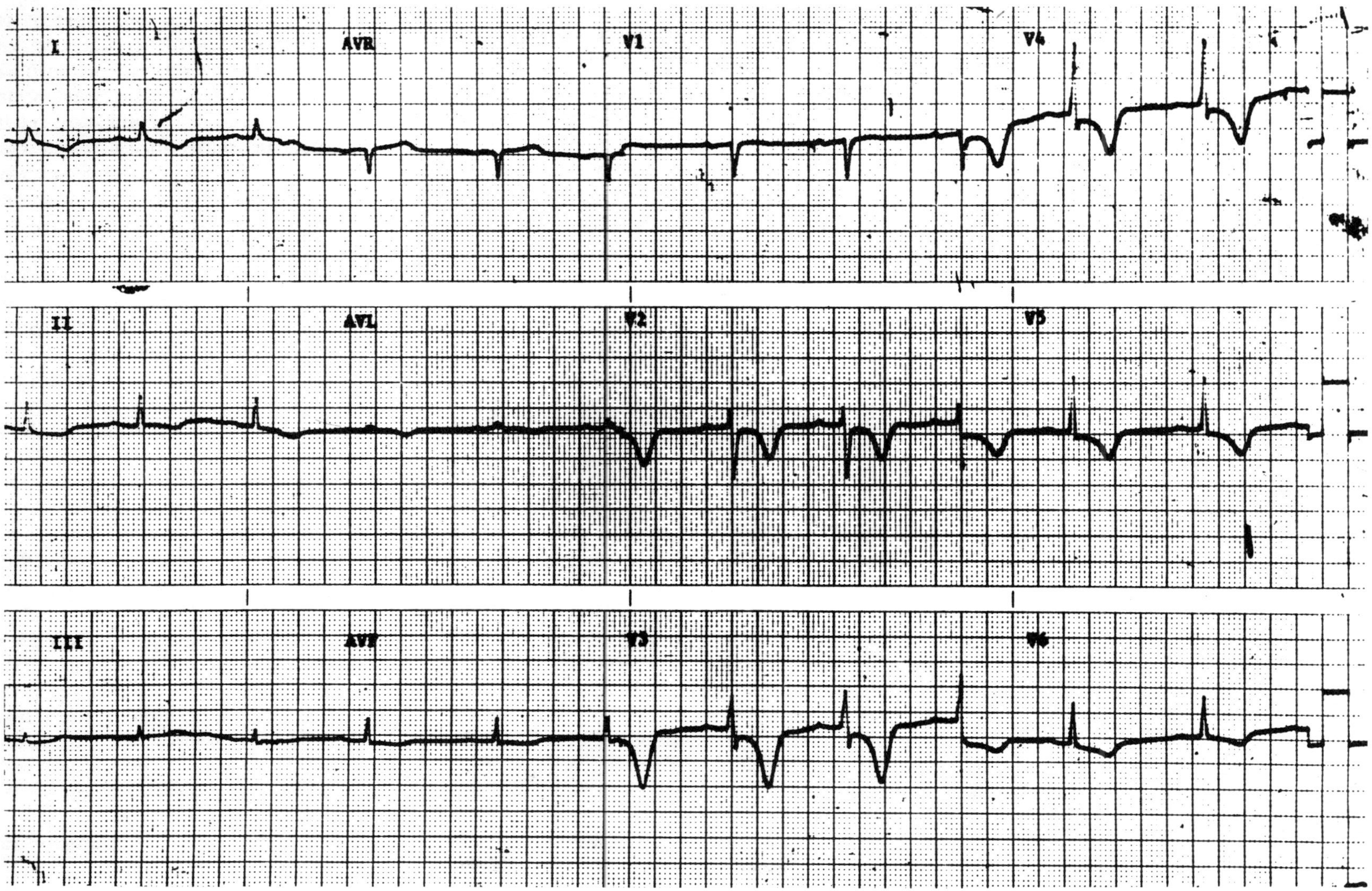


**Figure 47** A 62-year-old postal employee had the onset of acute substernal pain two hours prior to the admission electrocardiogram shown here.

# NUMBER 47 *Run Silent, Run Deep* Stephen P. Glasser, Pamela I. Clark

## ELUCIDATION

**Diagnosis**—*Subendocardial myocardial infarction*

The tracing demonstrates T-wave inversion across the precordial leads. No pathologic Q waves are present. Serial enzymes revealed a rise in CPK-MB, peaking 24 hours after the onset of pain.

## DISCUSSION

The electrocardiogram (ECG) is a useful method of diagnosing myocardial infarction when classic changes occur, but even in transmural infarction the ECG has limitations. In subendocardial infarction the ECG is even more unreliable in diagnosing infarction but, in addition, is unreliable in localizing, sizing, or characterizing the depth of necrosis. The diagnosis of subendocardial infarction is based more on the history of prolonged ischemic pain in conjunction with a rise in cardiac enzymes, particularly CPK-MB, than it is on the non-diagnostic S-T and T-wave changes seen electrocardiographically.

Clinically, subendocardial myocardial infarction has been a poorly defined entity which has usually been thought to be a mild, benign, uncomplicated heart attack. Recently, several concepts related to this infarction have undergone reevaluation. Pathologic studies have demonstrated that the absence of Q waves does not rule out transmural infarction, and subendocardial infarctions discovered at postmortem examinations have been found to be associated with abnormal Q waves visualized on the EKG. Because of this, some have suggested the terminology be changed from transmural and subendocardial to "Q-wave" and "non-Q-wave" infarction. A greater clinical similarity to patients with obvious transmural infarction (with its associated complications) has also been recently recognized. Indeed, several studies have suggested that many patients with subendocardial infarctions may suffer an early progression to transmural infarctions. Kossowsky et al observed transmural myocardial infarction in 37% of patients 3 to 21 days following hospitalization for subendocardial myocardial infarction, and Abbott found a similar incidence of arrhythmias and hemodynamic abnormalities in comparing patients with transmural and nontransmural infarctions.

The diagnosis of subendocardial infarction should no longer be considered the benign entity previously thought; rather, it should be considered a close associate of transmural infarction. The same careful therapeutic and diagnostic considerations apply to this subset of patients as they do to the general population of coronary disease patients.

## SELECTED READINGS

Abbott J: Non-diagnostic EKG in patients with acute MI. *Am J Med* 55:608, 1973.

Kossowsky W: Superimposition of transmural infarction following acute subendocardial infarction. *Chest* 69:758, 1976.

Madias J: The myth of acute "mild" myocardial infarction. *Ann Intern Med* 86:347, 1977.

4. Stimmel B, et al: Q wave development in acute subendocardial MI. *Arch Intern Med* 131:676–678, 1973.

# NUMBER 48 *A Heart Matter or the Gallbladder?* Stephen P. Glasser

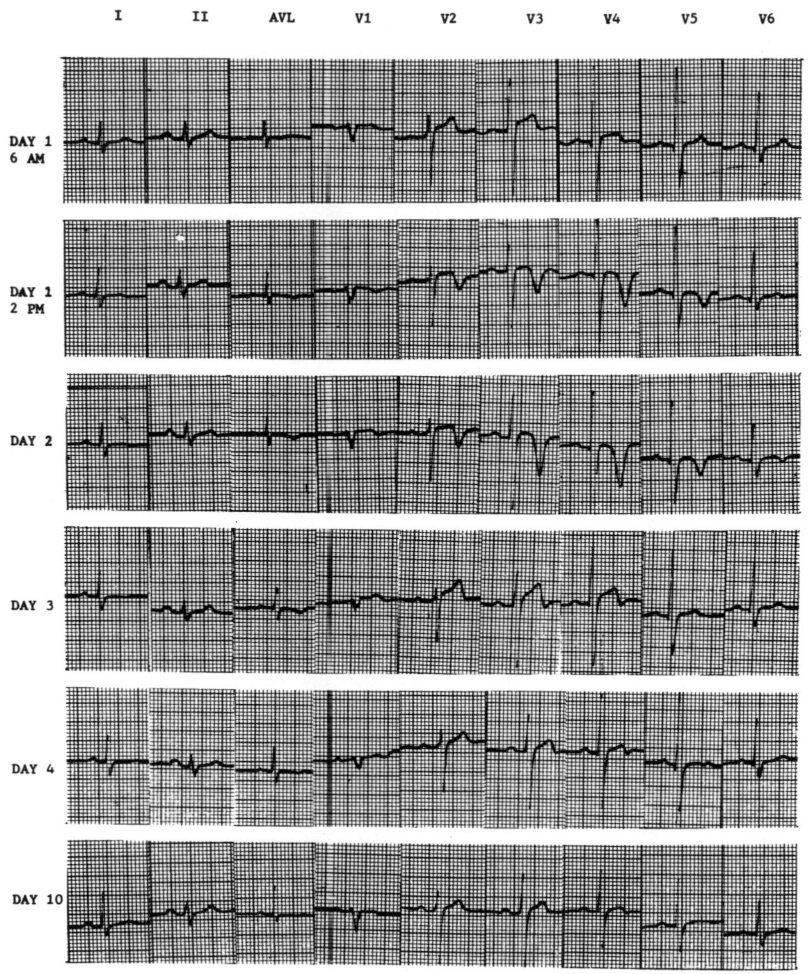


**Figure 48** A 54-year-old farmer was completely asymptomatic until three days prior to admission when he developed lower sternal heaviness after eating. On the day of admission, the pain persisted for four hours, radiated to the right shoulder, and was associated with dyspnea and diaphoresis. Intramuscular Meperidine was given two hours prior to admission. The only significant physical finding was a prominent apical $S_4$. The chest x-ray was normal. Serial electrocardiograms are shown, and serial enzymes were equivocal. Did this patient have a myocardial infarction or acute cholecystitis?

# NUMBER 48 *A Heart Matter or the Gallbladder?* Stephen P. Glasser

## ELUCIDATION

The main changes occur in the mid-precordial leads and suggest the evolution of an anterior wall, subendocardial, myocardial infarction. However, gallbladder disease is known to result in pain simulating myocardial infarction in association with ST-T wave changes. A technetium pyrophosphate scan was positive, suggesting the former diagnosis.

## DISCUSSION

A similarity in symptoms of gallbladder and coronary artery diseases was noted as early as 1878. Subsequently, changes in the ST segments and T waves in association with gallbladder disease were observed. Hodge distended the gallbladder or common bile duct at surgery in 26 patients with biliary disease. Disturbances in rate, rhythm, and T waves were noted, although not to the degree seen in coronary disease. Glotzer however, did note ST-T changes identical to those occurring with myocardial ischemia during traction of the gallbladder. Finally, others have noted electrocardiographic improvement in ST-T waves after gallbladder surgery. Kaufman and Lubera also demonstrated reversion of marked ST-T wave changes to normal in three patients with gallbladder disease when atropine was administered. Because of this, they suggested that the mechanism was reflex coronary artery spasm. As these studies took place before the era of coronary arteriography, the mechanism of these changes remains speculative.

## SELECTED READINGS


Breitwieser ER: Electrocardiographic observations in chronic cholecystitis before and after surgery. *Am J Med Sci* 213:598, 1947.

Glotzer S: The effect of traction of the gallbladder on the electrocardiogram. *NY State J Med* 55:515, 1955.

Hodge GB: The electrocardiogram in biliary tract disease and during experimental biliary distention. *Surg Gynecol Obstet* 86:617, 1948.

Kaufman JM, Lubera R: Preoperative use of atropine and electrocardiographic changes. *JAMA* 200:109, 1967.

## NUMBER 49 *2:1 Wenckebach* Stephen P. Glasser

LEAD II

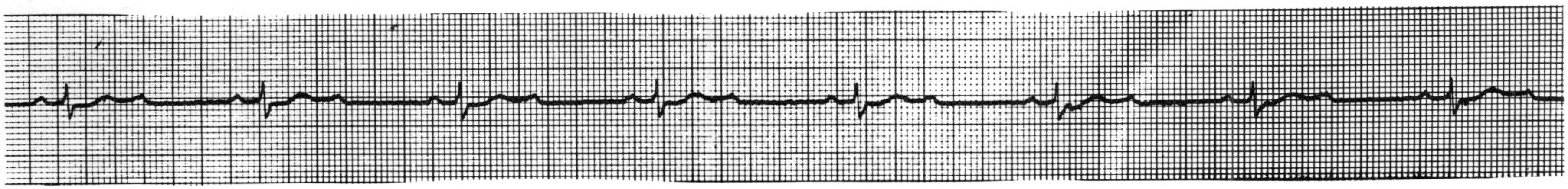

LEAD II

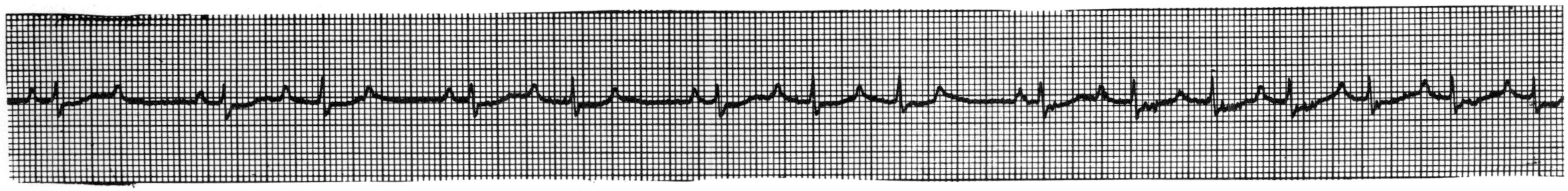

**Figure 49-1,2** This electrocardiogram was obtained from a 70-year-old woman with recent onset dyspnea and fever. A left lower lobe pneumonitis was present. Further history revealed that the patient had been placed on a "tablet" one week prior to be taken on a TID basis for two days and then once per day thereafter. Because she was not feeling well, however, she continued taking the medication three times daily. Her BUN was 70 mg/dl.

## NUMBER 49 *2:1 Wenckebach* Stephen P. Glasser

### ELUCIDATION

The rhythm strip demonstrates second-degree atrioventricular (AV) block which had been interpreted elsewhere as a Mobitz type II heart block. The conducted beats occur at a PR interval of 0.20 seconds. The interval P wave does not conduct. The P-P interval is constant at 0.70 seconds. Further history revealed that the "tablet" taken by the patient three times daily was digoxin. Because of this, 0.6 mg of atropine was administered intravenously during ECG monitoring. Shortly thereafter, the rhythm strip seen in Figure 49-2 was recorded. This demonstrates a rather classic 3:2 Wenckebach periodicity (Mobitz I block).

### DISCUSSION

If 2:1 block predominates (particularly if the conducted QRS complexes are normal in duration) the distinction between type I and II may be difficult. Since it is well known that digitalis causes block at the AV node, it was suspected that the rhythm strip depicted in Figure 49-1 was a 2:1 Wenckebach (type I) AV block. Long rhythm strips with close observation and the use of atropine will, in the majority of cases, reveal the transition to longer Wenckebach periods, allowing for a distinction in the two types of second degree block.

## NUMBER 50 *Rapid Atrial Stimulation for the Conversion of Arrhythmias*

Mallan G. Morgan, Stephen P. Glasser

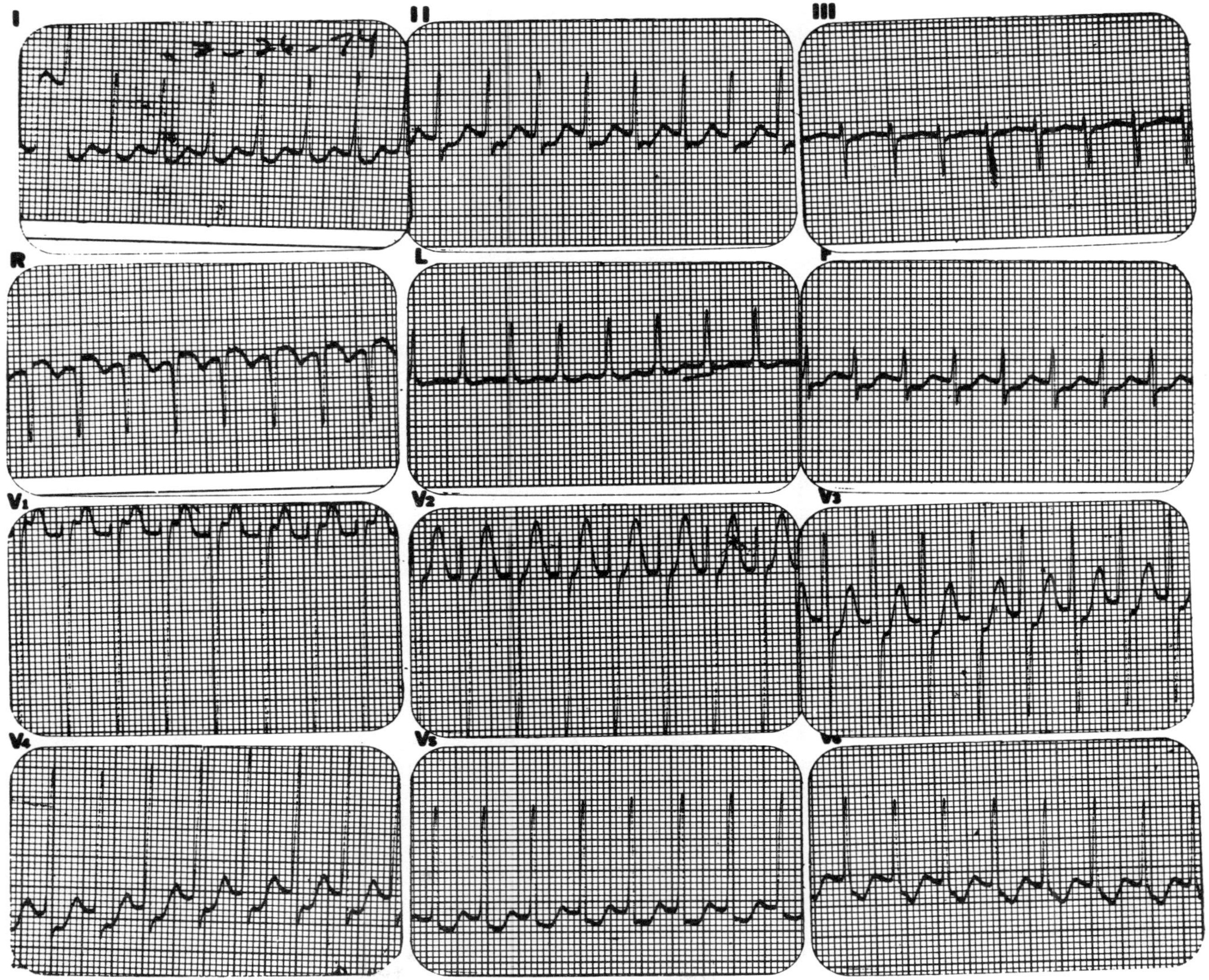


**Figure 50** This electrocardiogram was obtained from a 54-year-old woman with a history of bronchial asthma and palpitations.

# NUMBER 50 *Rapid Atrial Stimulation for the Conversion of Arrhythmias*

Mallan G. Morgan, Stephen P. Glasser

## ELUCIDATION

A supraventricular tachyarrhythmia at a rate of 200 is present. Distinct P waves are not seen. There is rather diffuse ST-segment depression suggesting ischemia. The most likely diagnosis is atrial tachycardia.

## DISCUSSION

This arrhythmia proved to be unresponsive to vasopressor therapy, edrophonium, quinidine, and digitalization. Propranolol was not given because of asthma. All cardiac stimulant drugs were discontinued, and electrical cardioversion was administered to a dose of 150 joules. This also failed to terminate the arrhythmia. The patient was then taken to the cardiac catheterization laboratory where atrial electrical stimulation was begun. At a stimulation rate of 220, transient atrial fibrillation occurred which then spontaneously converted to a normal sinus rhythm at a rate of 92. No complications ensued, and the patient has since been free of further episodes of atrial tachycardia while being maintained on cromolyn sodium, digoxin, and quinidine.

Paroxysmal supraventricular tachycardia is seldom fatal or even productive of severe symptoms except when prolonged or when it occurs in association with underlying cardiac disease. The attacks can usually be terminated by using the appropriate vagal maneuvers and antiarrhythmic drugs. For the occasional patient who does not respond to these procedures, normal sinus rhythm can be achieved with DC cardioversion. When there is a contraindication to DC cardioversion (digitalis toxicity or suspected toxicity) or there are frequent recurrences that necessitate multiple countershocks, rapid atrial pacing has been recommended and perhaps is the treatment of choice. Although there has been some controversy over the role of rapid stimulation in the conversion of atrial flutter, the use of right atrial pacing to convert atrial tachyarrhythmias (other than atrial fibrillation) is generally accepted, and there have been no known complications except in cases with anomalous AV conduction.

The mechanisms by which rapid atrial stimulation converts supraventricular tachycardias are probably either one or a combination of any of the following: 1) overdrive of an ectopic supraventricular pacemaker focus with resulting suppression; 2) conversion to another supraventricular arrhythmia (ie, atrial flutter to atrial fibrillation) for which conditions do not permit self-perpetuation; and 3) interruption of fixed circus movement. The most likely mechanism of the arrhythmia in this patient is that of a rapid-firing ectopic focus. This can be indirectly assumed from the atrial stimulatory rate that resulted in conversion of this patient's arrhythmia (ie, it implies overdrive suppression of an ectopic focus). Further documentation, of course, would have required programmed stimulation, which was not performed. In all of the reports to date, rapid atrial stimulation has been used when DC cardioversion was impractical.

This patient is unusual in that she proved refractory to all possible drug therapy as well as DC cardioversion, but was easily converted to sinus rhythm by rapid atrial stimulation. Our experiences with her would seem to suggest that in certain circumstances rapid atrial pacing might not only be preferable to DC cardioversion, but might also be the only effective treatment. The major disadvantages are, of course, related to the fact that rapid atrial stimulation is an invasive procedure and requires a certain amount of sophisticated equipment, and should be performed only by those experienced in the introduction and placement of intracardiac catheters and by those equipped to handle cardiovascular emergencies.

## SELECTED READINGS


Cheng T: Atrial pacing: its diagnostic and therapeutic applications. *Prog Cardiovasc Dis* 14:230–247, 1971.

Escher D: The treatment of tachyarrhythmias by artificial cardiac pacing. *Am Heart J* 78:829–832, 1969.

Haft JI: Treatment of arrhythmias by intracardiac electrical stimulation. *Prog Cardiovasc Dis* 16:539–568, 1974.

Lister J, Cohen L, Bernstein W, et al: Treatment of supraventricular tachycardias by rapid atrial stimulation. *Circulation* 38:1044–1059, 1968.

## NUMBER 51 *On the QT* Stephen P. Glasser

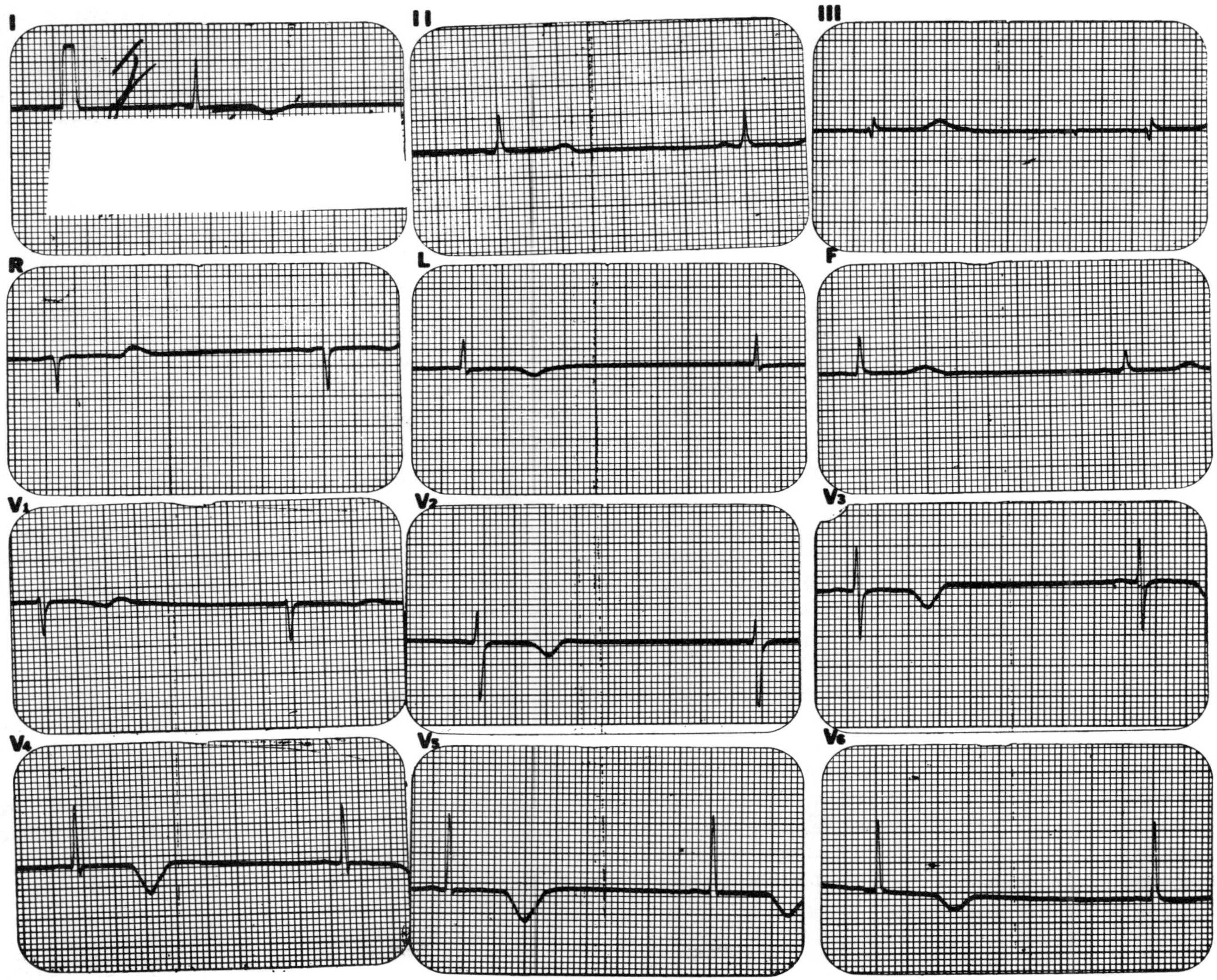


**Figure 51** The patient was a 19-year-old girl with diabetes insipidus.

# NUMBER 51 *On the QT* Stephen P. Glasser

## ELUCIDATION

There is a marked sinus bradycardia with a prolonged QT interval even when corrected for rate (QT = 0.60 second, QTc = 0.48 second). The QT prolongation is due primarily to a prolongation of the ST segment. This is characteristic of hypocalcemia and can be observed in chronic renal insufficiency, inadequate calcium intake, vitamin D deficiency, idiopathic hypoparathyroidism, partial or total parathyroidectomy, osteomalacia, respiratory or metabolic alkalosis or, as in the case of this individual, calcium loss. Although less common, flattening or inversion of the T waves may be observed. Significant cardiac arrhythmias are rare.

## DISCUSSION

"On the qt", according to the *Partridge Dictionary of Slang and Unconventional English,* means quiet. Perhaps this expression is appropriate when applying it to the QT interval since this interval is frequently overlooked in ECG interpretation. The QT interval is measured from the beginning of the QRS complex to the end of the T wave and represents electrical depolarization and repolarization of ventricular systole. It should be measured in a lead in which it is the longest and shows the termination of the T wave distinctly. This interval is affected by heart rate, becoming shorter as the rate increases, and therefore should generally be rate corrected. The best accepted formula for this is QTc = QT as measured/R-R, with the upper limit of normal being 0.405 seconds.

The principal effect of alterations in the serum calcium is seen in the ST segment and differentiates QT prolongation from quinidine effect, hypokalemia, etc. This is because calcium exerts its most prominent effect on phase 2 of the action potential, that phase most critically related to the ST segment on the surface ECG. On the other hand, phase 3 is relatively unaltered so that the T wave is unaffected. These effects are related to the concentration of ionized rather than total calcium so that one cannot necessarily relate the duration of the ST segment and the degree of hypocalcemia, although a closer correlation can be obtained if cerebrovascular fluid calcium concentration is measured.

Finally, it should be recalled that the effect of calcium on various electrophysiologic properties of the heart may be dependent upon the serum potassium concentration. Thus, intraventricular and atrioventricular conduction, and the facilitation of ventricular fibrillation caused by an increased extracellular potassium concentration, can be reversed or prevented by increasing the calcium concentration.

## SELECTED READINGS


Cobb TC: The QT interval. Progress notes. *Brooke Army Med Cen J* 10:39, 1967.

Lepeschkin E, Surawicz B: The duration of the Q-U interval and its components in electrocardiograms of normal persons. *Am Heart J* 46:9, 1953.

Surawicz B: Relationship between electrocardiogram and electrolytes. *Am Heart J* 73:814–834, 1967.

## NUMBER 52 *P on U* Stephen P. Glasser

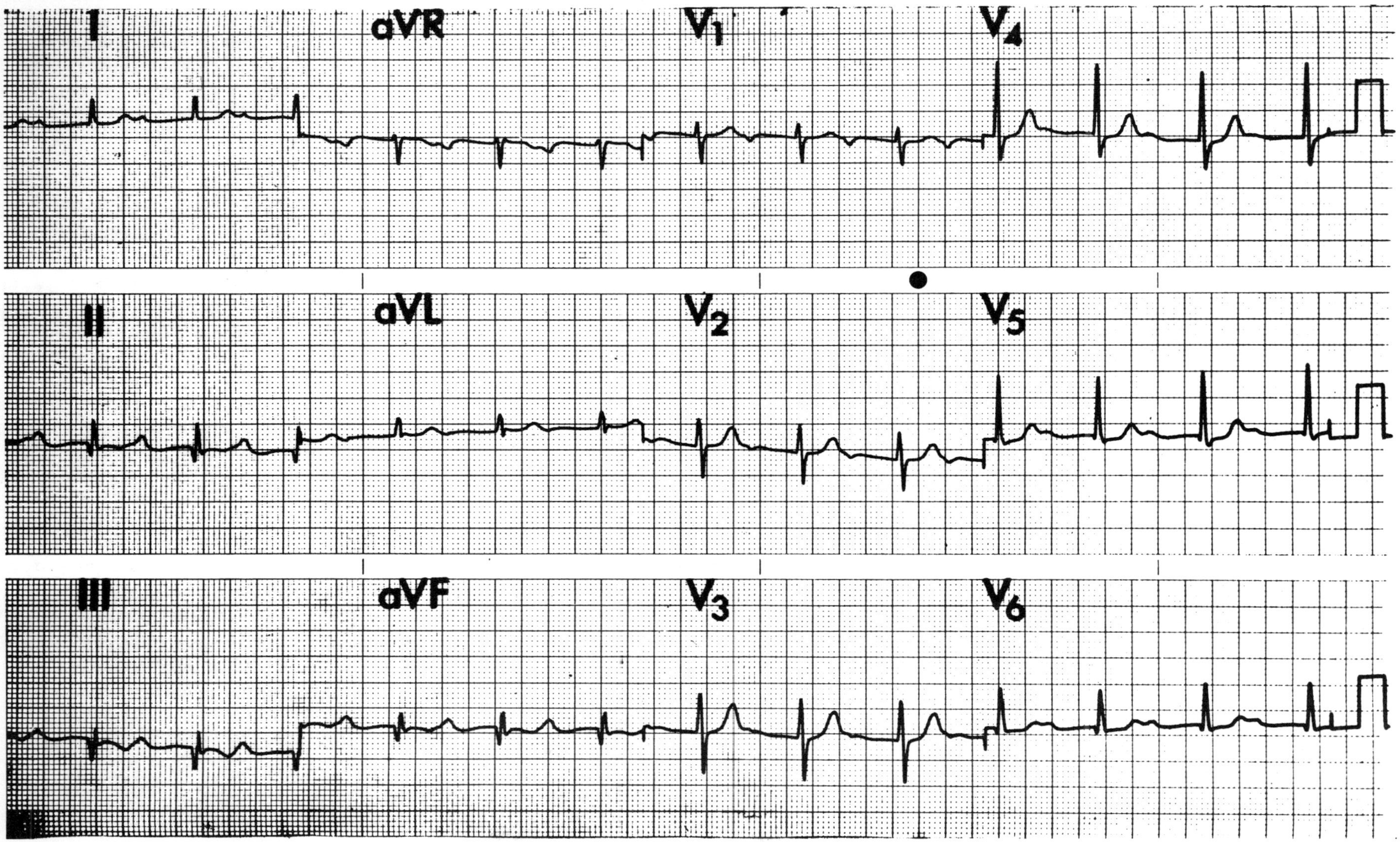


**Figure 52** This electrocardiogram was recorded from a 47-year-old man.

# NUMBER 52 *P on U* Stephen P. Glasser

## ELUCIDATION

The rate is 80, and the PR interval measures 0.42 second, consistent with first degree atrioventricular block. There are some ST-T wave changes present and the changes of a prior diaphragmatic myocardial infarction. The block had been present since an infarction one year before.

## DISCUSSION

When AV conduction is unusually prolonged or the R-R interval is shortened (ie, tachycardia), the conducting P wave can be either misinterpreted as a U wave or be obscured by an existing U wave, and this thereby defines the "P on U" syndrome. Junctional rhythm or hypokalemia can then be erroneously deduced. Also, with exercise, the U wave may become superimposed on the following P wave and P-Q segment leading to a false impression of S-T segment depression. Careful analysis of the U wave, T-P, and P-Q segments at slower heart rates may be necessary.

The U wave is the only waveform in the electrocardiogram whose genesis still remains controversial. The two major hypotheses generally accepted are that the U wave is due to the development of negative after-potentials in the ventricular myocardium or that the U wave represents repolarization of the Purkinje system. Delayed repolarization of certain portions of the ventricles has been a third, less generally accepted, theory. Normally, the U wave has the same polarity as the T wave but only 5% to 50% of its amplitude. It is highest in leads $V_2/V_3$ where it averages 0.33 mm, but may reach 2.0 mm in height. In general, U wave voltage varies directly with the T-wave voltage and to a lesser extent with QRS voltage, and is largest at slow rates. It is generally accepted that conditions which accentuate the U wave include hypokalemia, hypothermia, bradycardia, and quinidine administration.

A negative U wave has been observed with variable frequency in cases of hypertension, right and left ventricular hypertrophy, and myocardial ischemia. Negative U waves have been seen in up to 23% of hypertensives, and in some cases the U wave becomes positive with lowering of the blood pressure. Finally, a case of U wave alternans related to hypomagnesemia has been reported.

## SELECTED READINGS


Bashour T, Rios JC, Gorman PA: U wave alternans and increased ventricular irritability. *Chest* 64:377–379, 1973.

Lepeschkin E: The U wave of the electrocardiogram. *Mod Concepts Cardiovasc Dis* 39:45, 1969.

Watanabe Y: Purkinje repolarization as a possible cause of the U wave in the electrocardiogram. *Circulation* 51:1030–1037, 1975.

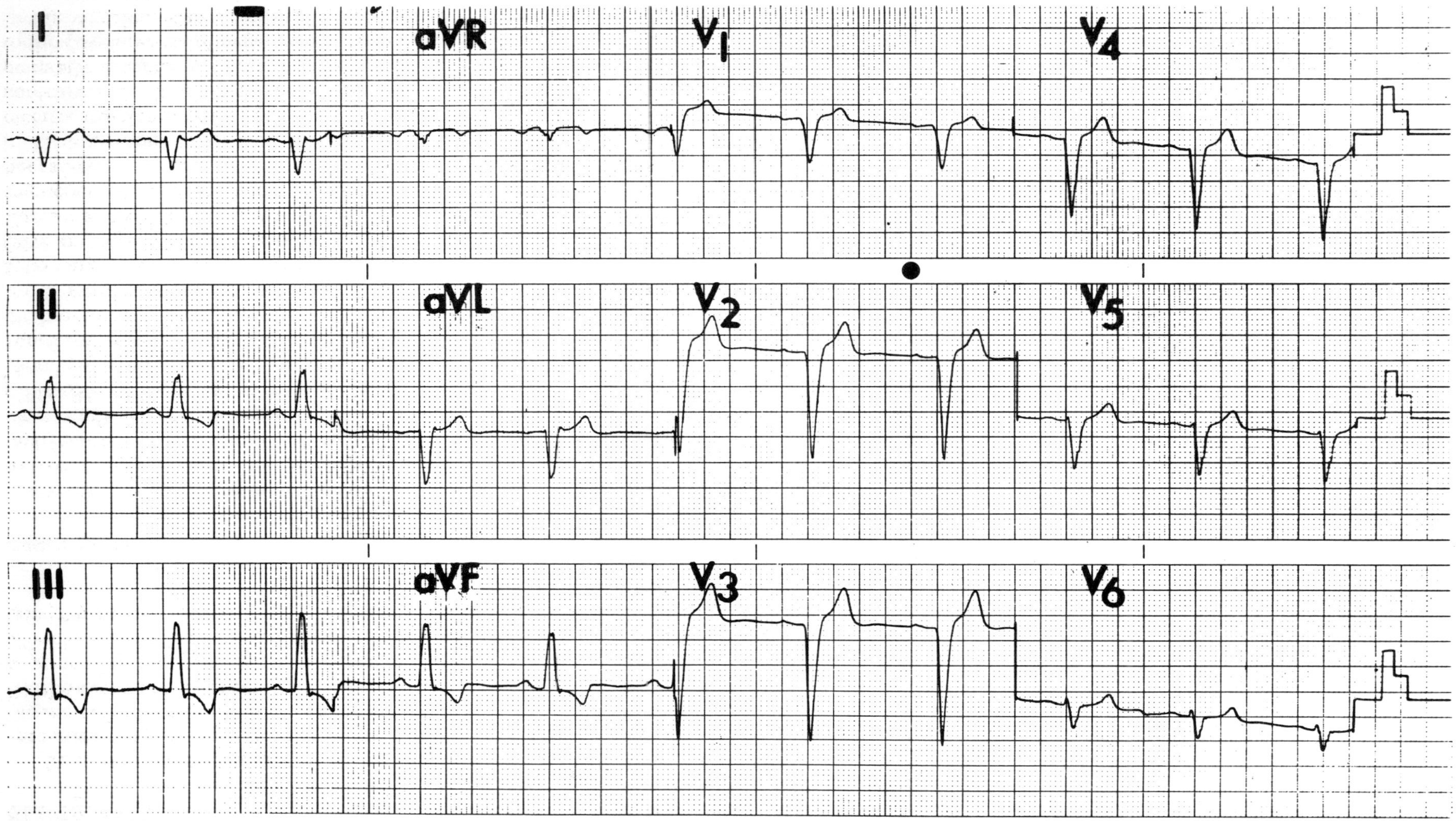


**Figure 53** This ECG was obtained from an 68-year-old asymptomatic man. No prior tracings were available for comparison.

# NUMBER 53 *Bundle Branch Block: Pre- or Post-Divisional?* Stephen P. Glasser

## ELUCIDATION

Complete left bundle branch block is present with a frontal plane QRS axis of +120. The PR interval is 0.18 to 0.20 seconds. The QRS width is 0.12 to 0.14 seconds.

## DISCUSSION

The concept of the trifascicular nature of the human intraventricular conduction system now has strong clinical, experimental, and histopathological support. Although the presence of right bundle branch block does not interfere with the diagnosis of either left anterior (LAH) or left posterior hemiblock (LPH), the electrocardiographic criteria of complete left bundle branch block (CLBBB) with additional block in the divisions of the left bundle branch system are less well documented.

Zakauddin et al demonstrated that with the appearance of CLBBB the mean frontal plane QRS axis was shifted to the left in 67 of 98 cases (a range of 2 degrees to 160 degrees), shifted to the right in 20 patients (a range of 3 degrees to 75 degrees), and did not change axis in 11. From this they concluded that an ECG prior to the development of CLBBB is helpful in evaluating the importance of the frontal plane QRS axis, ie, it seemed unlikely that these patients developed simultaneous predivisional LBBB and LPH or LAH, but that these changes in axis were consistent with CLBBB alone. There is nothing, of course, to say that these cases did not represent divisional LBBB with greater involvement in the anterior or posterior left bundle system. Lev et al studied the conduction system of eight cases of clinically diagnosed LBBB. They found no difference in lesions of the left bundle branch between cases with and without left axis deviation. They also found two factors involved in the mechanism of LBBB: a mechanical factor as evidenced by involvement of the summit of the ventricular septum, and that of ischemia of the left bundle as evidenced by severe three-vessel narrowing in five of the cases. DePasquale and Bruno suggested with clinical evidence that a QRS axis of −30 degrees or greater was not reliable evidence for block within the left anterior fascicle concomitant with main LBBB. Dhurandhar and Pickron presented a similar tracing in the ECG of the Month of the American Heart Association—Louisiana, Inc. and cited three conditions in which this unusual pattern could be seen:

1. Cardiomyopathy.
2. Extensive anterior wall infarction.
3. Chronic pulmonary disease and/or kyphoscoliosis associated with LBBB.

The significance of the right axis deviation in the case of LBBB reported herein is not definitely known, but may represent a concomitant left posterior hemiblock. With the borderline first degree AV block it was felt that His bundle electrography was indicated, but the patient refused study.

## SELECTED READINGS


DePasquale NP, Bruno MS: Left bundle branch block and abnormal left axis deviation without left anterior hemiblock. *Am J Cardiol* 32:98, 1973.

Lev M, Unger PN, Rosen KM, et al: The anatomic substrate of complete left bundle branch block. *Circulation* 50:479, 1974.

Zakauddin V, Gungor E, Tsung OC: Left bundle branch block with intermittent right axis deviation. *Am J Cardiol* 30:896, 1972.

## NUMBER 54 *Mispaced Placer or Misplaced Pacer* Stephen P. Glasser, Pamela I. Clark

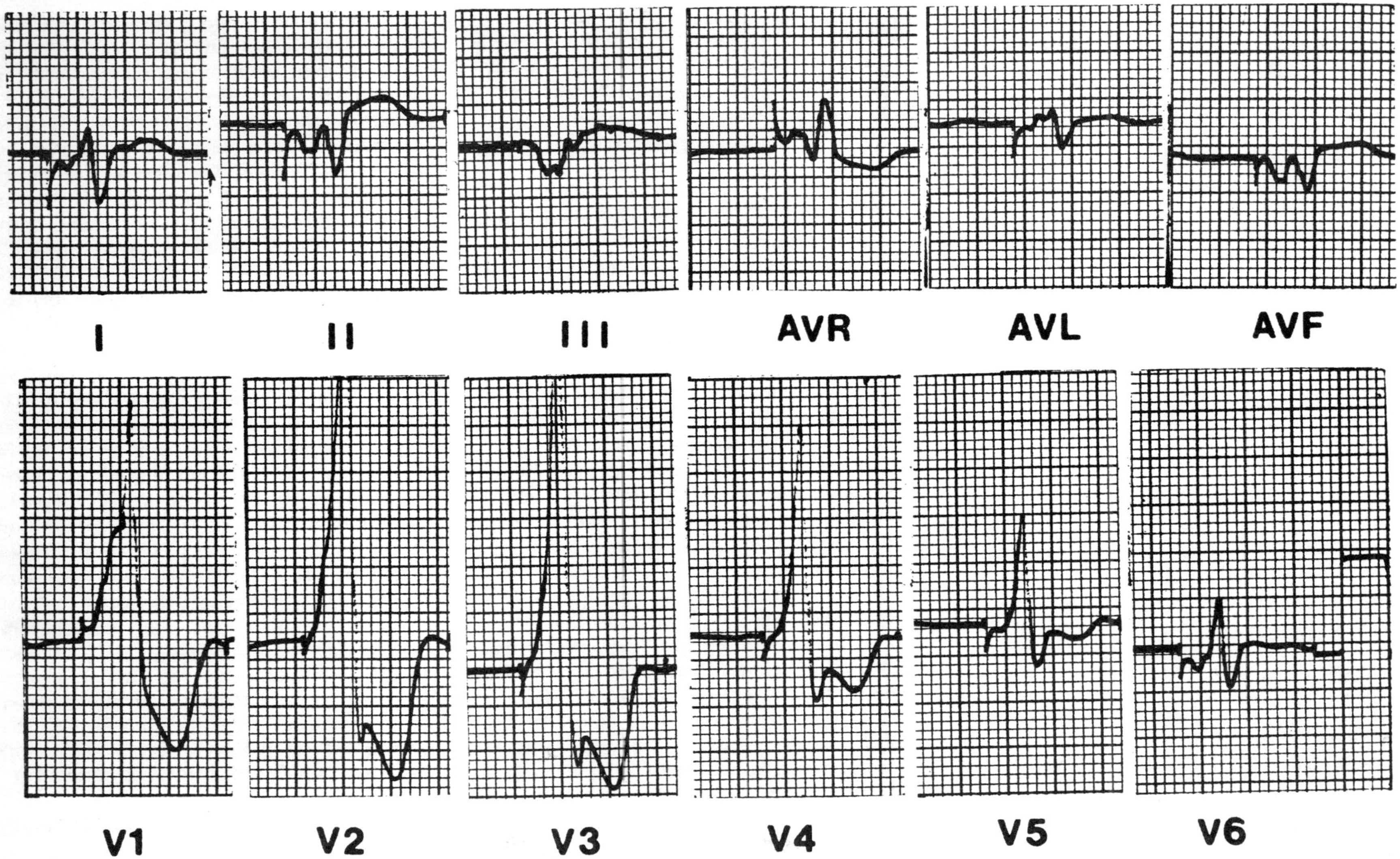


**Figure 54** This ECG is from a 66-year-old man with a permanent transvenous pacemaker, a holosystolic murmur, and cardiomegaly. Does the tracing lead you to believe that the pacemaker wire has been placed incorrectly (mispaced placer) or has it migrated to an inappropriate area (misplaced pacer)?

# NUMBER 54 *Mispaced Placer or Misplaced Pacer* Stephen P. Glasser, Pamela I. Clark

## ELUCIDATION

The ECG shows pacemaker spikes, each followed by a QRS of right bundle branch block (RBBB) configuration. We would expect a transvenous pacemaker to produce a LBBB complex because the left ventricle would be depolarized late. The RBBB pattern in this case indicates that the left ventricle is being activated before the right ventricle. This can be seen during pervenous pacing if the catheter is inadvertently placed in the coronary sinus (stimulating the left ventricular epicardial surface), if the right ventricle is perforated and the catheter migrates to the left ventricular epicardial surface, or if the pacemaker wire has perforated the intraventricular septum (or crossed a VSD). Rarely, an apparently well placed pacer can yield a RBBB pattern.

## DISCUSSION

By far the most common cause of RBBB pattern during presumed right ventricular endocardial pacing is malposition of the pacing catheter in the coronary sinus. Diagnosis is best confirmed by chest x-ray. A posteroanterior view of a pacemaker electrode properly positioned in the right ventricular apex will show the catheter to be to the left of the spine and close to the inferior surface of the heart. Placement in the coronary sinus may simulate apical pacing on a PA film, but a lateral view will show the catheter tip to be posteriorly directed, lying closer to the spine than to the sternum.

Catheter perforation of the right ventricular free wall is a less common cause of RBBB. If the extracardiac catheter tip lies in contact with the epicardial surface, capture will continue at a reasonable threshold, but usually capture soon ceases. Further manifestations of catheter perforation include friction rub or stimulation of the diaphragm or intercostal muscles. Perforation is accompanied by surprisingly low morbidity. Bleeding around the catheter into the pericardium is usually scant, and withdrawal of the electrode into the right ventricle generally does not lead to tamponade. Greatest morbidity is probably related to failure to capture.

Perforation of the intraventricular septum is a very rare cause of RBBB pattern during transvenous pacing. The man whose ECG is shown in Figure 54 had a holosystolic murmur which had been heard at a young age. The possibility of a congenital VSD was entertained, but cardiac catheterization confirmed the pacemaker position in the coronary sinus, no evidence of VSD, and cardiomyopathy with mitral regurgitation.

## SELECTED READINGS


Furman S, Escher D: *Principles and Techniques of Cardiac Pacing.* New York, Harper & Row, 1970, p 180.

Richards AM: Coronary sinus pacing masquerading as intraventricular septal perforation by transvenous catheter. Reply to Drs Cheng and Castellanos. *Am J Cardiol* 26:548, 1970.

# NUMBER 55 *A Message in Massage* Stephen P. Glasser

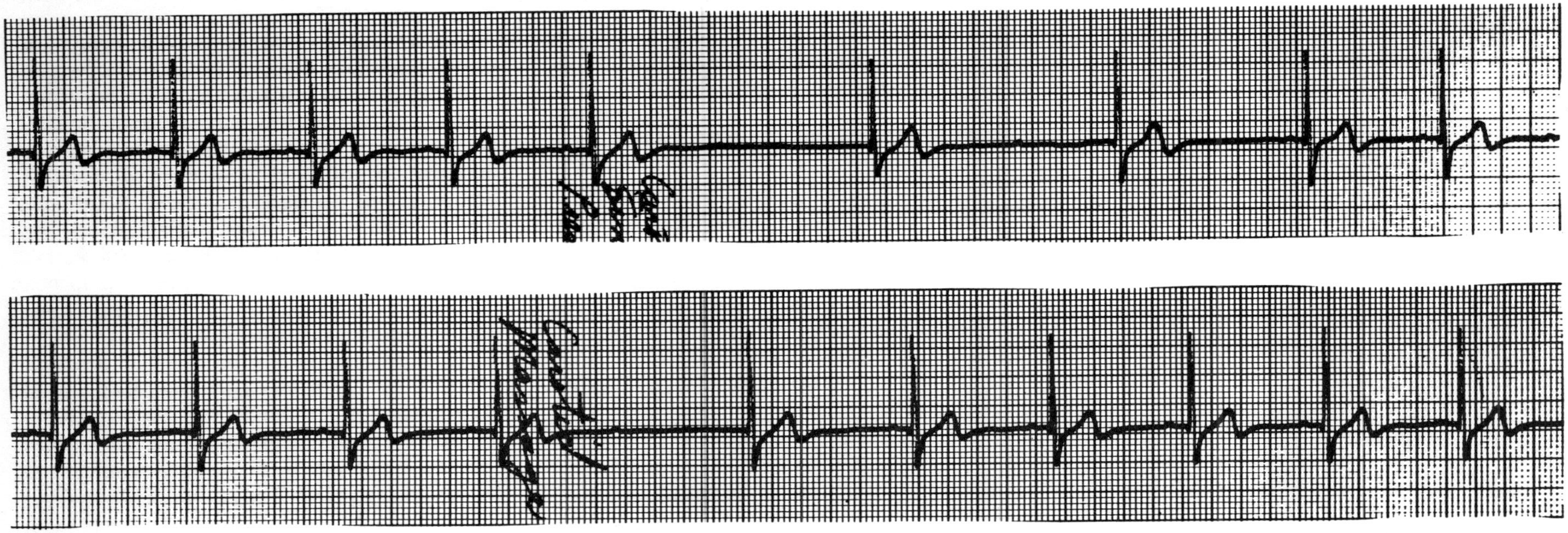

**Figure 55** The lead II rhythm strip in this figure shows two sequences of carotid massage in a 57-year-old man with dizzy spells.

## NUMBER 55 *A Message in Massage* Stephen P. Glasser

### ELUCIDATION

With carotid massage there is either marked sinus slowing or sinus arrest. Also present are blocked P waves (arrows) which are followed by junctional escape beats.

### DISCUSSION

Carotid sinus stimulation is generally associated with either moderate slowing of the sinus rate or sinus arrest. However, also reported are atrioventricular block, PR prolongation, and complete asystole. Carotid sinus sensitivity is generally considered to be present when postcarotid stimulation cardiac asystole lasts three seconds or more and is associated with a decrease in systolic and diastolic blood pressure of 50 mm Hg or more. In 1974, Glasser et al reported a case in which carotid sinus stimulation produced block at the atrioventricular junction as documented by His bundle electrography. In that study, His bundle electrography and sinus node recovery time were further utilized to document the presence or absence of sinoatrial or atrioventricular conduction disease. In the case presented above, one can see slight PR prolongation in the 5th beat of the top strip with the onset of carotid massage. This is followed by a P wave which is blocked, presumably at the level of the AV node. A junctional escape beat follows.

Carotid sinus massage has also been advocated as a provocative test for the sick sinus syndrome in the belief that the pause following this maneuver is suggestive of inappropriate sinus node responsiveness and sinus node disease. This is in contrast to the belief that the abnormality is one of excessive vagal input into a normal sinus node. Although not settled, such a response should at least alert the physician and would suggest further investigation.

Because of the patient's recurrent dizzy spells and in spite of a normal sinus node recovery time following rapid atrial stimulation, a pacemaker was placed. The patient has remained asymptomatic since the last follow-up visit. This case again demonstrates the usefulness of carotid sinus massage and points out some of the more unusual responses possible.

### SELECTED READINGS


Glasser SP, McCarty RN, Iannone LA: Hyperactive carotid sinus reflex and His bundle electrography. *J Electrocardiography* 7:71, 1974.

Lown B, Levine S: The carotid sinus. *Circulation* 23:766, 1961.

Parks K: Electrocardiographic findings following carotid sinus stimulation. *Ann Intern Med* 13:270, 1939.

Scarpa WJ: The sick sinus syndrome. *Am Heart J* 92:648, 1976.

Thomas JE: Hyperactive carotid sinus reflex and carotid sinus syncope. *Mayo Clin Proc* 44:127, 1969.

# NUMBER 56 *LVH?* Stephen P. Glasser

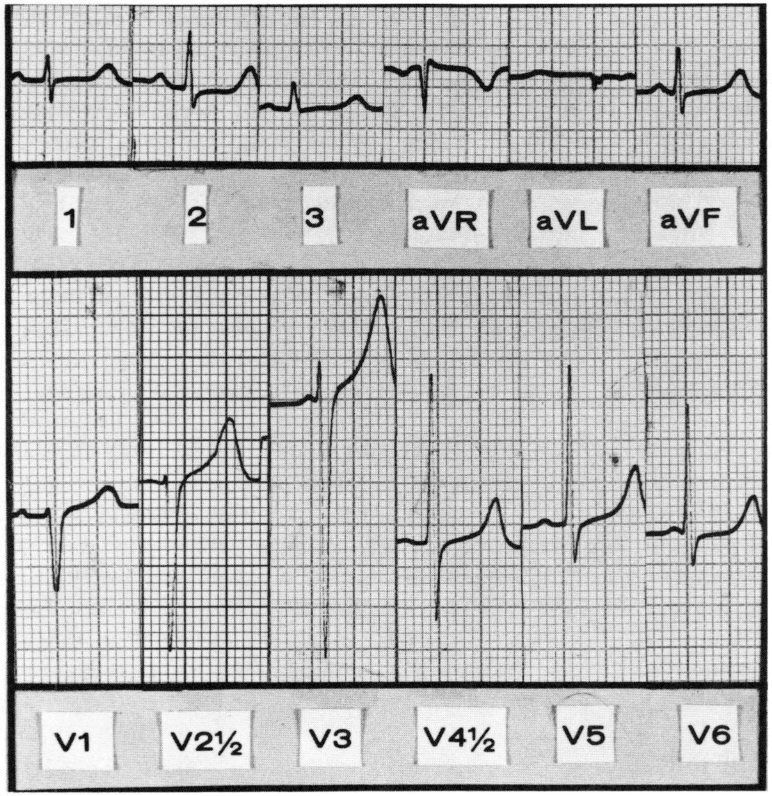


**Figure 56-1** The patient was a 20-year-old man.

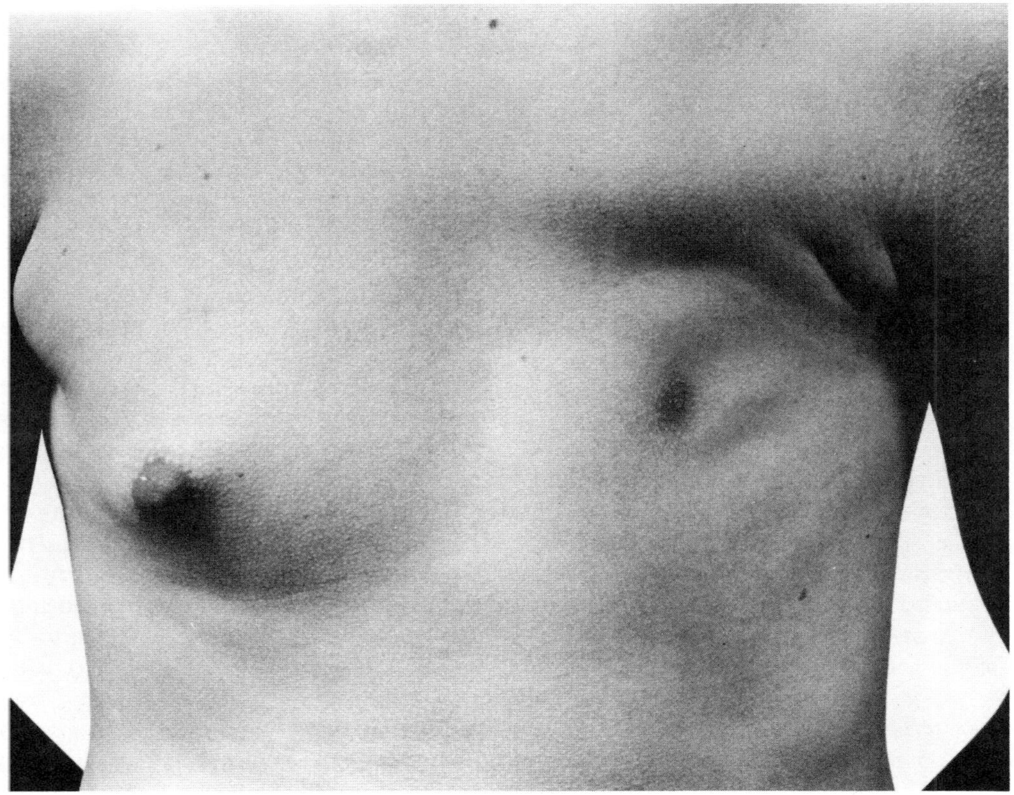

**Figure 56-2** Congenital absence of the left pectoral muscle.

## NUMBER 56 *LVH?* Stephen P. Glasser

### ELUCIDATION

The electrocardiogram is highly suggestive of left ventricular hypertrophy. However, physical examination revealed congenital absence of the left pectoral muscle (Figure 56-2).

### DISCUSSION

There are many extrinsic as well as intrinsic factors that must be considered when one is rendering an electrocardiographic diagnosis. Changes in the electrocardiogram have been reported after left and right mastectomy, in emaciated individuals, and with age. It is well known that body build must be taken into account in the electrocardiographic interpretation.

LaMonte and Freiman reported changes in the P, QRS, and T waves after right and left mastectomy (mostly radical procedures). They found large increases in the QRS complexes over the entire precordium (but not in the limb leads) after left mastectomy. The leads showing the most significant changes were $V_3R$ and $V_1$–$V_3$. After right mastectomy, significant increases in the amplitude of the QRS complexes were noted in $V_3R$ and $V_1$. They concluded that after mastectomy the standard criteria for electrocardiographic diagnosis may not apply and that after any alteration in the composition or configuration of the thorax, standard criteria should be employed with caution.

Numerous criteria for the ECG interpretation of LVH have been proposed. Most are based, by necessity, on hearts obtained from autopsy cases of older individuals. It has been appreciated that more liberal voltage criteria should be applied to individuals in the younger age groups, but the exact criteria have not been agreed upon. The patient in the present report met several of the voltage criteria for LVH. Perhaps the most widely accepted voltage criterion for the LVH is that of Sokolow and Lyon which consists of $SV_1$ or $SV_2$ + $RV_5$ or $RV_6$ greater than 35 mm. In this patient it measured 59 mm. Wilson et al suggested the criteria of $SV_1 > 24$ mm.

It is the intent of this report to once again emphasize that the electrocardiogram is influenced by many factors other than intrinsic heart disease, and that its interpretation must be performed in the light of clinical history and physical examination. In this case, the ECG abnormality could be linked to the absence of the patient's pectoralis muscle. This entity is apparently distinctly unusual, and in Gray's anatomy only a brief mention of this condition is made. It is stated that "Deficiency or absence of the sternocostal part (of the pectoralis major muscle) is not uncommon. Absence of the clavicular part is less frequent. Rarely the whole muscle is wanting."

Although no other cardiovascular lesions were noted in the case reported, it has been said that absence of the pectoralis major is sometimes associated with absence of the breast in females or other abnormalities of the cardiovascular system.

### SELECTED READINGS


Chou TC, Booth RC, McWhorter HB: Specificity of the current electrocardiography criteria in the diagnosis of left ventricular hypertrophy. *Am Heart J* 60:371, 1960.

Grant RP: *Clinical Electrocardiography.* New York, McGraw-Hill Book Co., 1957.

LaMonte CS, Freiman AH: The electrocardiogram after mastectomy. *Circulation* 32:746, 1965.

Walker CHM, Rose RL: Importance of age, sex, and body habitus in the diagnosis of left ventricular hypertrophy from the precordial electrocardiogram in childhood and adolescence. *Pediatrics* 28:705, 1961.

Wilson FN, Johnston FD, Rosenbaum FF, et al: The precordial electrocardiogram. *Am Heart J* 27:19, 1944.

## SELF-ASSESSMENT SECTION

### Educational Objectives

Following completion of this program of continuing medical education, the learner may take the following examination.

As an organization accredited for Continuing Medical Education, Louisiana State University School of Medicine in New Orleans certifies that this program of continuing medical education meets the criteria for 15 credit hours in Category 1 for Educational Materials for the Physician's Recognition Award of the American Medical Association, provided it is completed according to instructions.

For 15 hours of Category 1 CME credit, answer the self-assessment questions on the tear-out answer sheet found on page 159 and forward with a check for $75 made out to

to: Office of Continuing Education
LSU School of Medicine
1542 Tulane Avenue
New Orleans, LA 70112

### Continuing Medical Education Quiz

1. Concerning right bundle branch block, all of the following statements are true *except:*

   a. In some cases a number of maneuvers (eg, inspiration, Valsalva, carotid sinus massage) can result in normalization of conduction.

   b. Tachycardia-dependent bundle branch block is more common than bradycardia-dependent block.

   c. This conduction defect is more frequently associated with organic heart disease than with the absence of disease.

   d. The initial forces are not significantly altered so that the Q waves of infarction will not be masked.

2. Regarding subendocardial myocardial infarction (SEI), which statement best applies?

   a. The ECG changes in SEI are reliable indicators of the size of infarction.

   b. The diagnosis of SEI is more dependent upon history and enzymatic changes than it is upon the ECG changes.

   c. SEI generally represents a benign condition with good long-term prognosis compared to transmural infarction.

   d. At autopsy, transmural infarction is unlikely to be found unless Q waves were present on the ECG during life.

3. Which of the following is a *true* statement?

   a. Ventricular arrhythmias in the acute phase of myocardial infarction are good indicators of a poor long-term survival.

   b. Ventricular premature beats occurring after a long coupling interval are unlikely to provoke repetitive ventricular arrhythmias.

   c. Ambulatory monitoring has revealed that, in patients with coronary disease, S-T segment depression may occur with or without concomitant angina.

   d. The frequency response of ambulatory monitoring equipment is of no consequence in evaluating S-T changes.

4. Regarding Prinzmetal's angina which of the following statements best applies?

   a. During ambulatory monitoring S-T segment elevation is diagnostic of this syndrome.

   b. The diagnosis can be suspected by a history of nonexertional chest pain accompanied by S-T segment elevation.

   c. During ambulatory monitoring postural changes have no influence on the assessment of S-T segment shifts.

   d. During ambulatory monitoring the ability to record at least two precordial leads is of no advantage.

5. Which of the following statements best applies to second-degree heart block?

   a. In Mobitz I second-degree heart block the anatomic site of the block usually is above the bundle of His.

   b. Mobitz II second-degree heart block is usually a more benign condition than Mobitz I block.

c. Wenckebach (Mobitz I) heart block cannot occur in the bundle branches.

d. Group beating is classically seen in Mobitz II block.

6. Regarding the electrocardiographic changes in hypertrophic obstructive cardiomyopathy, which of the following statements best applies?

a. Atrial arrhythmias are common presenting manifestations.

b. Wolff-Parkinson-White syndrome is common.

c. Left ventricular hypertrophy is rare.

d. Q waves mimicking infarction occur in up to 25% of patients.

7. Which of the following statements is true?

a. A number of central nervous system diseases may produce striking ST-T wave abnormalities.

b. Certain arrhythmias are characteristic of central nervous system disease.

c. Most reported cases of T wave alternans suggest that this is a benign condition.

d. Sinoatrial block is almost always due to atherosclerotic heart disease.

8. Regarding carotid sinus massage which of the following statements is *not* true?

a. Massage of the carotid is usually associated with either moderate slowing of the sinus rate or sinus arrest.

b. Carotid sinus massage has been reported to cause complete asystole and transient atrioventricular block.

c. Carotid sinus sensitivity is generally considered to be present when post-carotid stimulation cardiac asystole lasts 1.5 seconds or more.

d. Carotid sinus massage has been advocated as a provocative test for the sick sinus syndrome.

9. Which of the following statements is true?

a. When a RBBB pattern occurs as a response to the paced rhythm of a right ventricular transvenous pacemaker, it should be presumed that pacemaker malposition has occurred.

b. The situation described in "a" is best diagnosed by a posteroanterior chest film.

c. The greatest morbidity from transvenous pacing is from catheter perforation of the right ventricular wall.

d. When a paced RBBB pattern occurs during transvenous pacing, it is diagnostic of pacer malposition.

10. Regarding ST-segment changes and/or T wave inversion, which of the following is *not* true?

a. Gallbladder disease is a cause of these changes.

b. Central nervous system disease has been associated with these changes.

c. Disturbances in rate and rhythm, and changes in the ST-T wave have not been noted during traction on the gallbladder or during bile duct surgery.

d. Technetium pyrophosphate scanning may help in the differential diagnosis.

11. Regarding the pre-excitation syndrome which of the following statements is true?

a. At least three bypass tracts have been related to this syndrome.

b. A short PR interval is diagnostic of a bypass tract.

c. A patient with a short PR interval and delta waves should be placed on antiarrhythmic agents even if asymptomatic.

d. The James bypass tract results in PR prolongation with QRS widening.

12. Atrial flutter is an often undiagnosed or misdiagnosed arrhythmia. Which of the following statements is *not* true?

a. Group beating in atrial flutter should raise the possibility of a Wenckebach phenomenon.

b. One-to-one atrioventricular conduction never occurs with atrial flutter because the A-V node is incapable of transmitting impulses at that rate.

c. Carotid sinus massage may be a useful technique in the diagnosis of atrial flutter.

d. Atrial flutter and atrial tachycardia have similar mechanisms of occurrence, with the atrial rate and P wave morphology acting as the main differentiating features.

13. Concerning bundle branch and fascicular block, which of the following statements is true?

a. LBBB is usually due to pre-divisional involvement of the left conduction system.

b. Left anterior (superior) fascicular block generally results in a right axis shift.

c. Conduction system disease resulting in intraventricular block is most often due to sclerodegenerative disease.

d. Left posterior fascicular block is a common condition generally resulting from atherosclerotic disease of the left anterior descending coronary artery.

14. Which of the following statements is most true?

a. A negative U wave on a resting ECG is virtually diagnostic of ischemic heart disease.

b. Sinoatrial block may be manifested as first, second, or third degree block.

c. Mobitz I (Wenckebach block) is characteristic by lengthening PR and R-R intervals.

d. S-T segment elevation in the immediate postinfarction period is highly suggestive of ventricular aneurysm.

15. A number of things affect the Q-T interval. Of the following, which is *least* likely to shorten or lengthen the true QT interval?

a. Sinus bradycardia.

b. Hypercalcemia.

c. Hypokalemia.

d. Hypocalcemia.

16. A number of mechanisms may be responsible for converting supraventricular tachycardias to sinus rhythm when utilizing the technique of rapid atrial stimulation. Of those listed below, which is the *least* likely?

a. Overdrive of an ectopic focus with resulting suppression of that focus.

b. Conversion to another supraventricular arrhythmia for which conditions do not permit self-perpetuation.

c. Changes in the hemodynamic status and hormonal changes (eg, sympathetic outpouring) resulting from this technique.

d. Interruption of a fixed circus movement.

17. All the following statements are true *except:*

a. Pericarditis may produce an atrial injury current manifested by a shift in the PR segment.

b. Mastectomy may produce increased QRS voltage.

c. 2:1 second-degree atrioventricular block may be due to Mobitz I (Wenckebach) block, and atropine administration may help to differentiate Mobitz I from Mobitz II block.

d. Mobitz I (Wenckebach) block is a dysrhythmia unlikely to be caused by digitalis intoxication.

18. Which of the following statements is true?

a. Rapid atrial stimulation for supraventricular tachycardia may be preferable to DC electrocardioversion when digitalis intake has been recent.

b. Changes in serum calcium affect primarily phase 3 and 4 of the action potential.

c. Arrhythmias are unlikely to be associated with ventricular aneurysm.

d. All of the above are false.

19. Which of the following statements is true?

a. The right bundle branch is supplied primarily by the right coronary artery.

b. The pattern of left posterior fascicular block may be mimicked by lateral wall infarction, acute cor pulmonale, or may occur in normal persons with vertical hearts.

c. Complete trifascicular block results in a normal PR interval with a wide QRS.

d. The occurrence of left anterior fascicular block is uncommonly associated with anterior infarction but, when they occur together, they portend a poor prognosis.

20. Which of the following statements is true?:

a. The refractory period of each conduction fascicle is directly proportional to the preceding cycle length.

b. The critical heart rate at which tachycardia-dependent bundle branch block occurs is generally higher for return-to-normal conduction than for the initiation of bundle branch block.

c. Intermittent RBBB is more likely to become permanent than intermittent LBBB.

d. The interpretation of ST-T wave changes is reliable in persons known to have intermittent LBBB.

21. Long-term ambulatory monitoring is becoming a more frequently utilized procedure in the evaluation of persons with proven or suspected heart disease. All of the following statements regarding this procedure are true *except*:

a. The frequency of arrhythmias has been shown to increase with the age of the individual tested.

b. It is generally the test of preference (compared to the resting ECG, stress testing, telemetry) in the evaluation of transient ST elevation of Prinzmetal's angina.

c. Good symptom and arrhythmia correlation has been reported in most studies in the literature.

d. The specificity for ST segment changes is in the order of 60%.

22. Which of the following ECG signs has *not* been associated with central nervous system disorders:

a. Prolonged QT interval.

b. T wave inversion.

c. Supraventricular arrhythmias.

d. Ventricular arrhythmias.

e. All of the above have been associated with CNS disease.

23. The "causes of pauses" on the electrocardiogram include all of the following *except:*

a. Sinus node arrest.

b. Wenckebach block.

c. Nonconducted atrial premature beats.

d. Interpolated ventricular premature beat.

24. Carotid sinus massage may be expected to be helpful in the evaluation of all the situations listed below *except:*

a. Atrial flutter.

b. Sick sinus syndrome.

c. Atrial tachycardia.

d. Ventricular tachycardia.

25. Deep precordial T wave inversion may occur in all of the following *except:*

a. Prinzmetal's angina.

b. Subendocardial myocardial infarction.

c. CNS hemorrhage.

d. Gallbladder disease.

26. Which of the following statements regarding accelerated idioventricular rhythm (AIVR) is incorrect?

a. It represents a sustained, active (by usurpation) ventricular rhythm.

b. It is *not* indicative of heart disease.

c. It is associated with transient AV dissociation.

d. It must be differentiated from ventricular tachycardia and junctional rhythm with aberration.

27. The most distinctive landmark on the electrocardiogram with extreme degrees of hypothermia is:

a. The Ashman phenomenon.

b. The Osborn wave.

c. The development of supraventricular and ventricular arrhythmias.

d. An infarction pattern.

e. None of the above.

28. Electrocardiographic changes observed in patients with central nervous system disease include:

a. Changes in the P wave.

b. Shortened P-R interval.

c. Changes in the T wave.

d. QT prolongation.

e. All of the above.

29. Following right ventriculotomy, complete right bundle branch block frequently appears. This change may be produced by:

a. Disruption of peripheral branches of the right bundle branch or its arborization.

b. Surgical trauma to the main right bundle.

c. Both *a* and *b*.

d. Neither *a* nor *b*.

30. Select the *incorrect* statement regarding chaotic atrial tachycardia:

a. Rarely, a ''benign'' variety has been observed in healthy young individuals.

b. It is usually unresponsive to digitalis and quinidine.

c. It cannot be confused with atrial fibrillation or atrial flutter with variable AV block.

d. Changing P wave morphology is characteristic.

31. Which is incorrect for the *U wave?*

a. Normally, it has the same polarity as the T wave.

b. Failure to differentiate the T wave from the U wave can lead to erroneous measurement of the QT interval.

c. Its inscription is likely related to the development of negative afterpotentials in the ventricular musculature.

d. Negative (inverted) U waves are virtually always associated with heart disease.

32. AV dissociation:

a. Is never a primary disturbance of rhythm.

b. Does not necessarily require therapy.

c. Can be observed in healthy individuals.

d. Is synonymous with complete AV block.

33. With regard to bidirectional tachycardia, which of the following is *not* true?

a. It implies a good prognosis.

b. Ventricular rate is in the range of 130 to 180 per minute.

c. It is often due to digitalis intoxication.

d. There is no universally successful single form of treatment.

34. The most common ECG changes associated with mitral valve prolapse are:

a. Prominent and inverted U waves.

b. Early repolarization changes with the precordial leads.

c. Nonspecific inferior wall ST-T wave changes.

d. Those of Wolff-Parkinson-White syndrome.

35. The blood supply to the SA node always comes:

a. Exclusively from the right coronary artery.

b. Exclusively from the left anterior descending coronary artery.

c. From either the right or left circumflex coronary artery.

d. Exclusively from the left circumflex coronary artery.

36. The sick sinus syndrome is:

a. Produced only by disease in the SA node.

b. Seen twice as often in men as in women.

c. Never a primary diagnosis.

d. Seen most frequently in individuals below the age of 50.

37. Which of the following is *not* characteristic of sick sinus syndrome?

a. Recurrent ventricular tachycardia.

b. Sinus bradycardia.

c. Paroxysmal atrial fibrillation.

d. Paroxysmal atrial flutter.

38. Which of the following is *not* characteristic of second-degree block at the AV node?

a. Narrow QRS complexes.

b. It is more common than second-degree block distal to the bundle of His.

c. It can occur only when the basic rhythm is sinus in origin.

d. It improves with atropine and exercise.

39. Mobitz type I AV block (Wenckebach) exhibits all but which one of the following?

a. Acceleration of the ventricular rate.

b. The R-R interval following the pause is always equal to the R-R interval preceding the pause.

c. The P-R interval progressively lengthens.

d. Successive P-R increments progressively diminish.

40. Which of the following is not an ECG feature of dextrocardia?

a. Inverted P waves in leads I and aVL, positive in leads II, III, aVR, and aVF.

b. P waves remain upright in the left precordial leads during sinus rhythm.

c. ''Mirror-image'' QRS complexes in lead I.

d. Progressive loss of R wave from right to left in the precordial leads.

41. The major components of an artificial cardiac pacemaker are:

a. The electrical generator.

b. The catheter.

c. The electrode attached to the catheter.

d. All of the above.

42. All of the following are true of the early repolarization syndrome except:

a. It is a normal variant.

b. Observed patterns simulate acute myocardial injury.

c. It is also associated with T wave changes and large amplitude R waves in lateral precordial leads.

d. It can be symptomatic and requires treatment.

43. All of the following are true for sinoatrial block except:

a. Careful examination of the P wave provides clues to the diagnosis of first-degree SA block.

b. Second-degree SA block may be impossible to differentiate on the ECG from sinus bradycardia.

c. In third-degree SA block, escape rhythms become the dominant pacemakers of the heart.

d. Management is dependent upon the cause.

44. In regard to cardiac pacing, which statement is incorrect?

a. The amplitude of the pacemaker spike is determined by whether a unipolar or a bipolar electrode catheter is used.

b. Right ventricular pacing produces a complete left bundle branch block pattern.

c. Abnormal left axis deviation in the frontal leads indicates that pacing occurs at the outflow tract of the right ventricle.

d. Paced beats may exhibit retrograde ventriculoatrial conduction.

45. The presence of one or more abnormally prolonged QRS complexes on the ECG should prompt the interpreter to discard:

a. Aberration.

b. Bundle branch block.

c. Pre-excitation.

d. Ventricular ectopy.

e. None of the above.

46. All of the following are true of parasystole except:

a. It can occur anywhere in the heart.

b. The parasystolic focus exhibits variable degrees of entrance and exit block.

c. It is characterized by fixed coupling intervals.

d. It can be best established by careful analysis of rhythm strips.

e. The parasystolic and the manifest rates are seldom equal.

47. In regard to parasystole, it is not:

a. A benign arrhythmia.

b. A manifestation of digitalis toxicity.

c. Associated with fusion beats.

d. Due to enhanced automaticity.

48. Which of the following statements is false?

a. Frequent ventricular premature beats (VPB) can occur in the presence or absence of heart disease.

b. VPB may or may not be associated with symptoms.

c. VPB never disturb the basic sinus rhythm.

d. A compensatory pause may or may not follow VPB.

49. Which of the following statements is false regarding massive accidental digitalis intoxication or as a suicidal gesture?

a. A serious and relatively frequent complication is hypokalemia.

b. Ventricular arrhythmias are absent in patients with no heart disease.

c. Presenting manifestations are cardiac and/or extracardiac.

d. Dialysis is useless in eliminating digitalis.

50. All of the following statements about retrograde ventriculoatrial conduction are correct except:

a. It may be partially or totally intact in complete anterograde AV block.

b. It can be associated with retrograde Wenckebach sequences.

c. The P wave resulting from retrograde conduction always follows the QRS complex.

d. It can be observed with ventricular premature beats, ventricular automatic beats, and during ventricular pacing.

## PLEASE CIRCLE CORRECT ANSWER

1. a b c d
2. a b c d
3. a b c d
4. a b c d
5. a b c d
6. a b c d
7. a b c d
8. a b c d
9. a b c d
10. a b c d
11. a b c d
12. a b c d
13. a b c d
14. a b c d
15. a b c d
16. a b c d
17. a b c d
18. a b c d
19. a b c d
20. a b c d
21. a b c d
22. a b c d e
23. a b c d
24. a b c d
25. a b c d
26. a b c d
27. a b c d e
28. a b c d e
29. a b c d
30. a b c d
31. a b c d
32. a b c d
33. a b c d
34. a b c d
35. a b c d
36. a b c d
37. a b c d
38. a b c d
39. a b c d
40. a b c d
41. a b c d
42. a b c d
43. a b c d
44. a b c d
45. a b c d e
46. a b c d
47. a b c d
48. a b c d
49. a b c d
50. a b c d

*(Please print)*

Name ______________________________

Address ______________________________

City ____________________ State __________ Zip ______